# Getting started in private practice

By Gene Balliett

Medical Economics Company 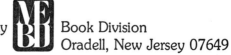 Book Division
Oradell, New Jersey 07649

*Design by JoAnne Cassella*

ISBN 0-87489-134-5

Medical Economics Company
Oradell, New Jersey 07649

First Printing      November, 1978
Second Printing      May, 1979

Printed in the United States of America

# Contents

(Continued)

# Publisher's notes

Gene Balliett is a medical management consultant, writer, editor, and lecturer. He has advised more than 600 physician-clients, coast to coast, on practice management and personal finances. Hundreds have attended his lectures for doctors and their spouses, and his workshops for business-office employees.

In addition to "Getting Started in Private Practice," his other books are "How to Close a Medical Practice," also published in the fall of 1978 by Medical Economics Company Book Division, and "The Business of Dental Practice," published by Professional Publishing Company in 1967. In the same year he contributed to Horace Cotton's classic, "Medical Practice Management" (first edition), also for Medical Economics Company.

Mr. Balliet joined Medical Economics magazine as a copy editor in 1962 after a seven-year newspaper career in Ohio and New York. As a senior editor of the magazine, he contributed to a series of articles on do-it-yourself practice check-ups that won a

Neal Award, the business magazine journalism equivalent of the Pulitzer prize.

He left Medical Economics magazine in 1967 to freelance and launch his own management consulting firm. From 1972 to 1975, he also served as editor of a practice management magazine for physicians. His writings since then include a regular practice management column for a biweekly news magazine for physicians, this book, and "How to Close a Medical Practice."

Mr. Balliett frequently conducts seminars and workshops for the nonprofit Seminars & Symposia, Inc.; Practice Management Association, Inc. of New York; the American Medical Association; and state and county medical and specialty societies. He is listed in Marquis' "Who's Who in America."

# Acknowledgments

In the mid-1960s I was a senior editor at Medical Economics, heading up the department that produced the practice management articles. That meant I dealt regularly with some of the country's best medical management consultants. Names such as Richard Bibbero, Oscar Gaarder, Roger Harrison, Millard Mills, Mark Myers, John Post, Paul Revenaugh, Clayton Scroggins, and Nelson Young come quickly to mind from those days. They were fascinating people. After watching them at work in doctors' offices and in their own seminars and workshops—they're very serious about their own continuing education—I concluded that what they did was far more interesting than what I did.

So I became one of them, not at all realizing how much I still had to learn. I continued to pick their brains. I was trained to do so—I'd been a journalism major, a newspaper reporter, and an editor. But more to the point, I had to do so to survive. And they put up with me, sharing their insights freely over the years.

Doctors and medical assistants added to my on-the-job eduation, too; the number of doctor-clients became fuzzy somewhere around the 600 mark. But mostly my debt of gratitude is to the nation's medical management consultants—early on, the grandfathers, as the founders of the major firms are sometimes called, and, more recently, the younger ones. You'll find some of them quoted in this book. I won't even attempt to name all those who've given me good information or ideas.

Most of them are, like me, members of the Society of Medical-Dental Management Consultants. If I were to dedicate this book—I won't, because I think book dedications are silly—I'd dedicate it to them. These days, I depend on them for my continuing education and for bright, fresh thinking.

Gene Balliett
Teaneck, N.J.
August, 1978

# Introduction

When it comes to class and comfort, you just can't beat a Southern country club. Lunch—with fine linen and silver service and, best of all, a view of rolling greenery from an open veranda—is almost reason alone for a Yankee to head southward, winter or summer.

My client, Fred Bodner, M.D., and I were leaving just such a country club after taking a midday pause from our quarterly management consultation. As we reached the parking lot and walked toward his Mercedes, Dr. Bodner, a family practitioner, sighed audibly, shrugged in little-boy-lost fashion, gave me a sly, sidelong glance, and, with a trace of the Devil's own shine in his eye, said, "Ah, well. I'm just *not* a very good businessman."

Lord, I do hate to hear that line.

If I had a dollar for every time a physician has used it, I'd *buy* a Southern country club, throw the members off the place, and live there. It's high time, I say, that doctors realize they speak those words not because they're confessing something but because they're *proud* to be lousy businessmen, to be viewed as people who are above crass commerce. Many seem to go out of their way to avoid knowledge of the business side of private practice.

Fred Bodner (and that, by the way, is not his real name) is an old client of mine, so it's fitting that I use his story to kick off my book. I'll talk with you here just about the same way I talk with him. If I speak freely now, maybe I can keep you from becoming a victim of some attitudes that have served your elder colleagues badly.

At the base of what's wrong is their absurd notion that private practice is something other than a business. Well, of course, it's a business! Anyone who earns his living through the production of goods or services is in business. That's nothing to be ashamed of. And if you're not convinced that tending patients is a commercial matter, just consider:

• Health-care costs, which accounted for 4.6 per cent of the nation's gross national product in 1950, equaled 8.3 per cent of the G.N.P. in 1975.

• In 1976 doctors' fees rose about five times faster than the non-medical-care components of the consumer price index.

• The fees of doctors in private practice rose 30.7 per cent between the end of Federal economic controls, in April 1974, and the end of August 1976, but the cost of all goods and services rose only 19.4 per cent in that same period.

• The yearly cost of health care, it is authoritatively predicted, will be $223.5 billion by 1980. National health insurance will add another $10 billion to $25 billion.

• In 1976 and 1977 Medicaid programs threatened to shrivel and shrink as major states, faced with continually rising payments for health-care goods and services, looked for ways to pull back from programs to provide health care for the poor, realizing that neither the poor nor the states can afford comprehensive health care. New York's Governor Hugh Carey, for instance, sought early in 1977 to end Medicaid reimbursement for a number of services, including physical therapy and private-duty nursing, while requiring the poor to come up with at least part of the money required for prescription drugs, eyeglasses, and dental care.

Because of the increasing price of health care, the American people have over the years warmed to the idea of national health insurance. But for the same reason, the Congress and the Democratic administration are having second thoughts about it. Can the United States find enough money to pay for comprehensive, cradle-to-grave health care? It probably cannot—not, at least, till it finds a way to exert some control over the costs.

Just what does lie ahead? Well, fee-for-service private medicine will surely continue. It's now thriving in Britain as an alternative to a national health system that has sputtered along from its inception. It continues to function freely in Canada, where fee-for-service practitioners bill the Government, rather than the patients, for most of the services rendered. And it will continue to thrive here, no matter what directions the Government health policy takes.

In time, I expect, even the Government programs will rely on fee-for-service compensation. Forget about capitation; it rewards shirking, rather than productivity, and some of our Federal health planners will see that soon enough. Though baiting bureaucrats is a popular pastime, the fact is that our Government does contain some bright, capable, well-trained people who are intent on getting a good job done. In the health sector, they probably will. After some false starts and pilot projects and new programs that chalk up few successes and many failures, they'll notice that medical practice is a kind of piecework industry, that some doctors perform lots better than others, and that fee-for-service compensation is a far better way of attracting the productive doctors than is capitation.

Both bureaucrats and lawmakers will eventually realize that many of medicine's wrongs either never existed or can be fixed easily. This basic realization will affect their concept of group practice. Doctors have clinically been in group practice all along, even if 90 per cent or so are still practicing in one-, two-, and three-doctor offices. Even solo practitioners refer patients to specialists and subspecialists who are better able to manage various diagnostic and treatment problems, and so all doctors who refer or are referred to are in a *de facto* clinical group. Never mind that the group doesn't practice under one roof. Never mind that it doesn't report its income and outgo on a single Federal income tax return. Roofs and tax forms have nothing whatever to do with the quality of health care. And the quality of the services rendered by present-day medicine is demonstrably good.

That's not to say that the system is as good as it should be or will be. For instance, doctors are in short supply both in the slums and in the sticks.

In the slums what's needed is, first of all, some broad, work-able socio-politico-economic programs. People there need income, jobs, hope. The best preventive medicine is economic well-being. From it arises better diet, safer and warmer shelter, less anxiety—better health. But slums and poverty are only a part of a larger problem—the cities. Slums will only grow worse until our cities work again. And they can. Good cities are more fun than suburbs, more convenient than the country. There's no shortage of people who wouldn't happily return to safe, exciting, wealthy, beautiful cities. They'll do it, too, when we have those kinds of cities—not sooner.

In the sticks there's also hope and a way out. Medical outposts are already cropping up there. In the future they will be everywhere, thanks to increased reliance on physician's assistants; nurse practitioners; physical therapists; sophisticated, computer-assisted diagnosis; and doctor-directed, TV-assisted examinations.

In time, there will surely be a national health-insurance plan, but it will be based, I believe, on the development of group prac-tices, often laymen-owned, that serve as a competitive alternative to traditional private practice. These laymen-owned practices will have to meet Government-imposed standards for fees and quality of care in return for seed money and long-term financing.

Increasingly, you'll have to compete with these laymen-owned, laymen-operated, Government-underwritten group prac-tices. Don't count on patients' preferring the doctor-run practices. Remember: They're the kind that the present grumbling is all about. Patients may come to prefer the ambience, the better management, perhaps the better quality of patient care, and surely the lower prices that they'll find in the alternative system.

And don't count on a boycott by doctors. If the laymen-owned groups compensate their doctor-employees on a salary-plus-bonus arrangement based on productivity, they'll recruit and keep good, productive doctors.

And don't count, either, on a continuation of the health bureaucrat's naive belief in huge, all-under-one-roof, distant, inconvenient-to-patients facilities. He'll see that there's merit in having doctors' offices scattered where people live. A group can put general practitioners, family physicians, internists, OBGs, pediatricians, and perhaps some others in satellite offices built for one, two, or three doctors. Management's new tools—on-line, real-time minicomputers linked by laser beam to central computers—are making such deployment simple, even when charts and financial records are centralized. And the cost is getting less almost by the month.

So the time is now for practitioners to stop that old I'm-a-lousy-businessman song and dance. The answer to higher health-care costs is better management, not fee increases. If you and enough other social-minded doctors see the management alternative in time, then private health care won't be priced out of the reach of both poor and middle-class patients alike, and doctor-owned, doctor-managed practices will survive.

Meanwhile, what about your own financial security? You can expect to have far more of it than your elder colleagues ever did. For all their fee increases, they're not nearly as financially well off as you may think. They've mismanaged their practices, they've been conspicuous consumers, and they've fallen prey to hokey investment swindles.

I'll fight for your right to be just as foolish, but I expect that you'll be far better off than they because of a series of retirement-plan laws, starting with Keogh in 1962. This body of retirement-plan laws has made it possible for almost every middle-class American to build a fortune through tax-sheltered savings and investments. You, my friend, were born at a good time.

Just consider the future of, say, a young medical office manager who's paid $240 a week. She can build an investment account of nearly a quarter of a million dollars in 25 years, or more than half a million dollars in 35 years. That's just at bank interest. It's the kind of financial future clearly visible to, say, a woman who starts working for a good employer at age 20, becomes his $240-a-week office manager at 25, and retires at 60.

Because of the retirement plan laws, many people, not just

doctors, have unprecedented financial security assured. And if your office manager stands to do so well, believe me, you'll do even better. Those new laws look after bosses, too.

Ever-improving practice management will also help you thrive. My Southern friend, Dr. Bodner, has become a believer and a past master of practice management. When he says, "I'm just not a very good businessman," it's because he knows I always bite. He also likes to tell his friends that he taught me everything I know, but I don't rise to that line; there's more truth in it than he knows.

We medical management consultants don't invent all the stuff we tell doctors. Mostly, we get it from observing smart doctors like Dr. Bodner and in skull sessions with each other.

So don't think everything you read here is original. Mostly it isn't, but mostly it's well-tested, and it works—as well it must, my friend, because you're in trouble. In their desperate attempts to cope with inflation and taxes, to live a better life, and to find long-range financial security, your elders have very nearly priced themselves out of the reach of all the patients in the lowest economic class and many of those in the middle class.

Now, just as public antagonism toward doctors threatens to grow to alarming proportions, here you come.

Well, you can't rely on fee increases as the magical solution to all financial deficiencies and anxieties. That day is gone—or soon will be. If you intend to be in private practice and to be there successfully, you'd better take an interest in the good, sound management of time and resources.

If you can learn to run a highly productive practice in a well-laid-out office, charge reasonable fees, assemble a good staff, stay up to date with your specialty, and be just as good a doctor as your abilities permit, then you'll earn the right to say you're a good doctor *because* you're a good businessman.

# 1

## How to tell if
## those offers you're getting
## make any sense

I was seeing clients in Los Angeles some time ago when an internist-client asked me to speak with a friend of his, a family practitioner I'll call Dr. Hill. I had three meetings with Dr. Hill. After the third, he decided to leave private practice and take an administrative job that had been offered to him by the research division of a major pharmaceutical company.

Dr. Hill had been in a severe state of depression, so diagnosed by his psychiatrist. Neither had recognized that a big part of his problem was simply that he hated every minute of his working hours. The fact that I did recognize the problem was anything but genius; just about any medical management consultant would have seen the problem right away and made the same recommendation. Every year since then, I receive a Christmas card from Dr. Hill, and he always writes a little note on the back of the card. The message is always the same, thanking me for pushing him into accepting what he's come to view as the greatest job in the world.

1

## Getting started in private practice

In Pennsylvania I was asked to do a practice survey by Dr. Wall, as I'll call a pediatrician who had come to dislike crying kids, demanding mothers, and private practice. I didn't even bother finishing the survey. Instead, I leveled with the guy. Today, Dr. Wall is an emergency-room doctor, works regular hours, makes enough money to live comfortably, has all the time off for travel that he feels he needs, and, best of all, finds deep satisfaction in coping with the challenges of trauma and the drama of dealing with the unexpected. Dr. Wall, like Dr. Hill, is delighted that I talked him into leaving private practice.

On the other hand, Dr. Morris (that's not his real name) never went into private practice. He wrote to me from Vietnam about a month before he was to be returned stateside, and he appeared in my office two days after being released from active duty, after having phoned ahead from California. He and his wife found themselves a room with a king-sized bed at the local Marriott hotel, and he and I spent three consecutive mornings in conversation at the side of the hotel pool. At the end of that time, he, too, was convinced that private practice just wasn't for him. He had seen enough trauma to last a lifetime; he wasn't sure that he could cope with much more. Today, he's a professor at a Southeastern medical school, lives in a comfortable house in a beautiful seaside community, and both he and his wife love their life there.

Some of my best work as a medical management consultant, in my view, has been getting people like Dr. Hill, Dr. Wall, and Dr. Morris to stay out of private practice. If that sounds like bad marketing of management consulting services, don't worry. Even if no more than 5 per cent of doctors in private practice ever hire a management consultant, there'll be more than enough work to keep scores of us busy. And like Drs. Hill, Wall, and Morris, I, too, require a certain amount of job satisfaction.

There's no better way for me to get it than to help a client find his or her niche. Like many of my clients, I'm not especially money-motivated; I'd rather count my wealth in units of satisfaction. So don't think for one minute that the purpose of this book is to steer you into private practice so that you can become some management consultant's paying client.

2

Let's take a few minutes out, then, to sample the pros and cons of some alternatives to solo private practice:

1. *A university*. The best article I've ever seen about a physician who'd given in to a long-felt yearning to leave private practice for teaching was written by Lyndon K. Jordan, M.D., in the December 8, 1975, issue of Medical Economics. Here are some excerpts:

"The transition to the academic community was reasonably smooth. . . . But a couple of the traditional department chairmen—those whose interests lay in research, writing, and teaching rather than in rendering primary care—remained aloof. Maybe they felt threatened by the fact that I'd actually been in practice. . . . So they weren't always willing to go along with my determined practical approach. . . .

"I quickly learned that confrontation is not the game to play in academia; at this altitude the stakes are high and saving face is as sacred as saving life. . . .

"I experienced many . . . headaches familiar to departmental chairmen: budget worries, scheduling problems, grant requests, teaching commitments, recruitment chores, endless staff meetings, planning sessions, resolving squabbles between the residents and the various specialty services. . . .

"Most of my time [was] taken up with administrative duties and strategy meetings. Too often [I] had to conceal my own feelings and concede to others. . . . My spirits flagged as I looked back on my practice in a rural community where I was really somebody . . . where my payment might be a ham or 100 ears of corn—but always gift-wrapped in gratitude. . . . I knew I had to return to private practice. . . . I handed in my resignation.

"The administration and faculty accorded me that subtle coolness reserved for a defector. . . . They found it hard to believe that someone could try the ivory-tower way of life and find it wanting."

Dr. Jordan then listed these observations on professional life at the university:

● The university "is not a single entity but is made up of individual fiefdoms, whose chiefs have private ambitions that collide both with each other and with the collective university goals."

**3**

## Getting started in private practice

- At the university, "you'll find very big men—with very big egos. They may not always accept you on your terms."
- The game at the university, "as in big business, is money. Your finest efforts will amount to nothing if you can't attract solid financial support for your department."
- "You'll spend your days teaching others how to practice rather than keeping your own medical skills honed. And your students won't always appreciate your efforts."
- "Becoming a small fish in the great academic pond may leave your own ego needs unsatisfied."
- At the university, there's "more political entertaining to be done, more night meetings, more out-of-town professional expeditions."

If none of those conditions bothers you, Dr. Jordan advised, "perhaps you do belong in academia. As for me, I've been back in private practice for more than a year now and I've never been happier." I'd add only that an increasing number of jobs at the medical schools seem to involve patient care.

Just to give you an idea of the kinds of jobs that have been advertised lately, I'll cite three excerpts from ads that appeared in The New York Times:

FIGURE 1-1 ════════════════════════════════════════

### Key Figures in a Typical Well-Managed Practice

|  |  | Your figures |
|---|---|---|
| Production | $143,700 | ———— |
| Collection ratio | .957 | ———— |
| Gross practice income | $137,500 | ———— |
| Overhead | $ 51,150 | ———— |
|    Assistant wages | $ 16,630 | ———— |
|    Rent, utilities | $ 7,700 | ———— |
|    Other | $ 26,820 | ———— |
| Physician compensation | $ 86,350 | ———— |
|    Salary | $ 66,400 | ———— |
|    Retirement plan | $ 16,600 | ———— |
|    Other fringe benefits | $ 3,350 | ———— |

● "INTERNIST/TEACHER: Board certified internist. Preceptor. Assist in developing ambulatory care curriculum. Salary negotiable. Superior benefits package."

● "THE DEPARTMENTS of pediatrics, internal medicine, and psychiatry are seeking full-time faculty."

● "ASSISTANT DEAN: to assist in the administration of programs in undergraduate and graduate health professions, education, and in biomedical research. Salary and benefits competitive and commensurate with experience."

2. *Industry.* Many physicians started finding their way into jobs in private industry in the early 1960s, when the Kefauver-Harris Act resulted in pharmaceutical manufacturers hiring more doctors to supervise the tests required by that law. Then in 1970 the Occupational Safety and Health Act increased the need for physicians in industry. And the Toxic Substances Control Act, dealing with environmental damage caused by chemicals and other substances, prompted industry to recruit still more physicians. And, as medical care has become an ever-larger part of employee-benefit packages, industry has hired more and more doctors to see employee-patients.

According to an article by William Abrams in The New York Times of November 28, 1976, Mobil Oil, for instance, had five physicians on its payroll to staff a complete outpatient clinic for 3,800 New York City employees.

Abrams found that there are about 4,000 full-time corporate M.D.s, half of them occupational medicine specialists who oversee "everything from employee health to industrial and product safety." Another 10,000 doctors have part-time jobs. About 1,200 physicians are in the pharmaceutical field, another 800 are insurance-company medical underwriters and claims consultants, and a relative handful are scattered in various other assignments. Merrill Lynch, Pierce, Fenner & Smith, for instance, has an M.D. securities analyst specializing in health-care stocks.

Increasing numbers of physicians are apparently attracted to industry, Abrams' study indicates. One of the physicians he quotes, Leon J. Warshaw, M.D., chief medical director for the Equitable Life Assurance Society of the United States, said: "I get calls every

**5**

week from doctors who are interested in a change. They want to get out of the rat race of private practice."

At the time of Abrams' report, several companies in the New York metropolitan area paid their industrial physicians an average salary of $35,000 to $65,000, depending largely on experience, with benefits—including health and life insurance, pensions, stock options, bonuses, and profit-sharing plans—adding "over 25 per cent to the value of total earnings."

To earn the equivalent of a $35,000 salary, a private practitioner needs to generate $76,700 worth of services in patient care. That's a busier practice than most first-year practitioners enjoy; production totaling $60,000 is a somewhat more reasonable expectation. On the other hand, $76,700 is only about 55 per cent of the production in a typical well-managed practice.

I'll use that term elsewhere in this book, so I'd better explain here and now that by "typical well-managed practice" I exclude from consideration many of the physicians whose earnings are included in the statistics gathered by governmental and many other sources. The exclusion of part-timers and other physicians with marginal practices accounts for the big difference between the figures I quote and the figures you've read elsewhere. Also, my statistics are based on doctor-clients' records and tax returns— figures shared with many other medical management consultants. I

FIGURE 1-2

## What the Right Corporate
## Retirement Plan Can Mean

| Years of investment | Annual return on investment | | | |
|---|---|---|---|---|
| | 6% | 8% | 9% | 15% |
| 30 | $1,389,575 | $2,061,658 | $2,532,522 | $9,577,180 |
| 25 | 958,639 | 1,315,583 | 1,550,881 | 4,486,871 |
| 20 | 639,154 | 814,809 | 923,907 | 2,071,176 |
| 15 | 402,298 | 478,685 | 523,459 | 924,765 |
| 10 | 226,699 | 253,074 | 267,693 | 380,715 |

Annual investment: $16,600, made in equal monthly installments of $1,383.33.

think it's reasonable to say that consultant-managed practices are well-managed or, at least, are better managed than private practices in general.

Physicians are attracted to industry by more than salary. How does a private practitioner's working life compare with an executive's? Frank X. Wamsley made the comparison in the October 18, 1976, issue of Medical Economics. He reported that a private practitioner's usual workweek is 60 hours, while an executive, according to a Fortune magazine study, works 56 hours a week. The executive takes off three weeks a year, the physician two—plus "another 13 days or so scattered throughout the year," said Wamsley.

Stature in the community is another matter, however. Physicians, though less highly regarded today than in the past, remain near the top of the occupational heap in terms of esteem; businessmen are near the bottom.

3. *A hospital.* If you're in training now or have just completed it, then you know better than I do what the life of the full-time doctor is in the hospital. But perhaps you've wondered what kinds of jobs are available in hospitals. Then you'll be interested in this sampling of ads that appeared in The New York Times:

● "INTERNIST/PEDIATRICIAN: Comprehensive clinic. Board eligible. Excellent salary and benefits."

● "GERIATRIC PROGRAM: Board certification or eligibility in internal medicine or family practice. Excellent salary and very liberal benefits."

● "INTERNAL MEDICINE: Medical/surgical unit of prominent psychiatric hospital. Salary $33,705 to $35,375."

● "INTERNIST: For outpatient medical facility with heavy geriatric orientation."

● "PSYCHIATRIST: Board certified. Good salary and fringe benefits."

● "PART-TIME: Board qualified or eligible internist or F.P. General medical clinic. 5 mornings per week."

● "SENIOR PSYCHIATRIST: Unit director in a creative hospital setting. Salary to $30s."

● "EMERGENCY PHYSICIAN: 200-bed general hospital. Mal-

**7**

practice insurance paid. Salary commensurate with experience."
• "ANESTHESIOLOGIST: 210-bed hospital. No OB. 5-county area of 300,000 population."

4. *A health maintenance organization.* In Medical Economics' issue of April 19, 1976, Louis R. Zako, M.D., a Michigan family practitioner, reported on his experience with a big-city health maintenance organization that aspired to national recognition as a model of what an H.M.O. should be. He had been in private solo practice for 11 years and liked the idea of being his own boss, but he was intrigued by the idea of getting in on the ground floor of Government medicine "before fee-for-service could no longer

FIGURE 1-3 ═══════════════════════════════════════

## Gross Practice Incomes of Major Specialties

| | |
|---|---|
| $201,000 or more | Allergy<br>Cardiology<br>Pathology |
| $176,000 to $200,000 | Neurosurgery<br>Orthopedics<br>Ophthalmology<br>Otolaryngology |
| $151,000 to $175,000 | Dermatology<br>Plastic surgery<br>Radiology<br>OB/Gyn<br>Neurology<br>General surgery<br>Internal medicine (general) |
| $126,000 to $150,000 | Anesthesiology<br>Urology<br>General practice<br>Thoracic surgery |
| $101,000 to $125,000 | Gastroenterology<br>Pediatrics |
| $100,000 or less | Psychiatry |

Figures are for calendar year 1976 and are specialty averages.

compete with this Federally subsidized brand of medical care." Once on the payroll, however, he found that the bureaucracy of prepaid group practice required a great deal of patience.

"When I needed a specialist—orthopedist, neurologist, urologist—I was told . . . the wait . . . was 8 to 12 weeks. . . .

"We wanted to offer health education, the very heart of an effective H.M.O., but there was no money available for audiovisual equipment. . . .

"Charts were constantly misfiled. Some of those I'd brought with me from my old practice are lost to this day. . . .

"The H.M.O.'s appointment phone center was run by five or six operators untutored in triage. . . .

". . . the time span on ECG readings . . . sometimes . . . took a week, sometimes two weeks . . . then . . . a full month. . . .

"I ordered a brain scan. There was no equipment. . . . My patient's condition turned stuporous, and I saw him failing while I fought for basic diagnostics. I discharged him and arranged for a private neurosurgeon to admit him to [another hospital]. . . . From then on . . . if such a patient required sophisticated care, I hospitalized him at [the other hospital].

" . . . it's my impression that a doctor who under fee-for-service will operate for six hours when he shouldn't will, when on salary, not want to operate for six hours when he should.

"Let the health planners call fee-for-service a nonsystem, a cottage industry. I call it U.S. medicine at its best."

In a companion article, Joseph Hess, M.D., the chairman of the department of family medicine at Wayne State University's medical school, added these words:

"I work in a university, and I know how a large bureaucracy works—namely, slowly. . . . It takes a very sophisticated management system to make the practice of medicine efficient and professionally satisfying. That's one of the reasons it's not easy to develop a large organization that employs physicians and keeps them happy the way a private practice does."

In an earlier Medical Economics article from January 20, 1975, pediatrician Sol Browdy, of Trenton, N.J., painted quite another picture:

## Getting started in private practice

"I'm aware that H.M.O.s are an anathema to the average doctor; perhaps if they were called prepaid health plans instead of health maintenance organizations, the prejudice would vanish. I'm aware, too, that the average fee-for-service doctor believes he's doing as much to maintain his patient's health as H.M.O.s do, with regular checkups, screen testing, and immunizations. But in comparison with a hospital-affiliated H.M.O. like ours, he almost certainly isn't."

He found five significant ways that his colleagues in the

FIGURE 1-4 =======================================================

## Gains and Losses in Charges in the Major Specialties

Four specialties showed major productivity gains (their charges, after adjustments for poverty and courtesy discounts, were up by 25 per cent or more from 1975). Nine specialties had good gains (up 5 to 24 per cent). Four held steady or recorded modest gains (up 1 to 4 per cent). And four had median survey figures of less than those for 1975.

| | |
|---|---|
| Major gains | Otolaryngology |
| | Cardiology |
| | Neurology |
| | Pathology |
| | |
| Good gains | Orthopedics |
| | General surgery |
| | General practice |
| | Plastic surgery |
| | Internal medicine (general) |
| | Dermatology |
| | Ophthalmology |
| | Neurosurgery |
| | OB/Gyn |
| | |
| Modest gains | Pediatrics |
| | Allergy |
| | Psychiatry |
| | Urology |
| | |
| Down from 1975 | Radiology |
| | Anesthesiology |
| | Gastroenterology |
| | Thoracic surgery |

primarily physician-managed Mercer Regional Medical Group practiced better medicine—less overprescribing, less unnecessary hospitalization, more thorough histories and physicals, better quality control, and fewer paperwork distractions. On the last point, he said: "One of the biggest benefits for doctors in the H.M.O. is that we're relieved of all the business paperwork. The receptionist does the billing and collecting, and the physicians never have to think about it."

5. *Government.* Those comments about involvement with bureaucracies also apply to government employment. But let's not carry on further about that. Instead, let's just sample some of the ads from The New York Times:

● "MENTAL HEALTH REGIONAL DIRECTOR: State Dept. of Mental Hygiene. Responsible for planning, coordination & delivery of mental hygiene services. Extensive professional experience in treatment of people with mental or developmental discords including alcoholism. 4 years management experience. State license. Certification. $43,952 + fringe benefits."

● "REGIONAL HEALTH SERVICES DIRECTOR: State Department of Correctional Services. Evaluate the quality and quantity of health-care delivery. Salary: $38,000."

6. *Private group practice.* Philip R. Alper, M.D., a California internist who often writes for Medical Economics, once spent eight years in a three-man partnership. After getting out and going into solo practice, he wrote an article for the May 13, 1974, issue in which he said that "solo practice is THE way to get the most satisfaction out of medicine. . . .

"My partners were outstanding physicians, our practice standards were very high. There was just one thing wrong—I felt that too much time and energy were wasted due to needless conflict. When it seemed that our differences of opinion never would be eliminated, I made up my mind to go on my own. . . .

"In a solo setup, management-labor relations are at their most basic level. The assistants have only one boss to please, and he's in constant communication with them. It doesn't take a committee meeting to decide whether the ECG cart should be mounted on wheels or not, or what the charge for a urinalysis should be. The

**11**

ease with which decisions are made results in less tension and a happier crew. . . .

"I had feared that night calls would bedevil me in solo practice, but I found there were actually fewer calls than before. Patients seemed to become protective of a man who's 'their doctor,' and they encourage him to take his time off and rest. As a result, they think twice before dialing.

"Another surprise was finding out that coverage was not at all hard to arrange when I wanted to go out or do something with my family. As for weekends, eight of us now rotate taking calls and covering for one another. . . .

"Expenses in solo practice are slightly higher than in group practice, so net income is slightly lower, too [but] being solo allows a doctor greater flexibility. For instance, I've changed office hours to suit myself alone. . . .

"Advocates of group practice can throw back quite a list of advantages to prove their points, and their validity is hard to question. I know from my own experience that many group advantages are indisputable, but I also know that the drawbacks are there, too."

Here are some ads from The New York Times for group practice doctors:

● "ALLERGIST, DERMATOLOGIST, OPHTHALMOLOGIST, ORTHOPEDIST, OTOLARYNGOLOGIST, UROLOGIST: Expanding group practice. Board certified or eligible. Partnership after 24 months."

● "M.D. OR D.O.: Open-minded, interested in applying innovative diagnostic & treatment procedures in holistic medical & psychiatric practice; nutritional, orthomolecular, biofeedback, psychotherapeutic & other medical modalities. Emphasis is on prevention. Join two psychiatrists in rapidly growing private office practice. Salary $35,000 to $60,000 + fringe benefits."

To most groups asking me how to recruit, I recommend a supergood retirement plan—the kind that offers a young doctor a realistic shot at a million-dollar nest egg in as little as 16 years—to complement a salary-plus-bonus arrangement based on productivity. The salary is a guarantee. The bonus depends on the new doctor's production. The salary gives him an income from his first day in practice. The bonus gives him the assurance that, though there's a floor on his earnings, there's no ceiling. If he turns out to be highly productive, he may earn more money than the senior doctor in the practice.

But that gives us this final alternative to solo private practice:

7. *Two-doctor practice.* The terms are the same, I usually tell the senior physician, whether he's looking for a second doctor as an early step toward group practice—that is, three or more doctors—or toward his own departure into retirement.

Unfortunately, though, most senior physicians do not offer a salary-plus-bonus deal. They just offer straight salary. That may be fine for a new doctor who's absolutely depressed about his ability to get much going in private practice and who feels that he'll be lucky just to earn the salary. But senior doctors aren't often looking to recruit that kind of beginner.

So the salary deal they offer isn't appropriate for the recruiting job they're trying to do. They want a producer, so they should offer a compensation deal that rewards production. Obvious? Apparently not. The standard offering for years has been a straight salary the first year, 30 per cent of the net practice income the second, then 40 and 50 per cent in the third and fourth years. I call that compensation based on tenure, and I hate it because it leads to all sorts of problems. The worst of them are competition for time off, lack of incentive to the new doctor to take a proprietary interest in building up his own share of the practice, and, almost inevitably, the breakup of the partnership.

So I usually try to change the senior doctor's thinking, whether he or the new physician is paying my fee. I've found that partners have trouble enough living with each other without embarking together in a little financial boat that's already been proved undependable. What terms should you look for? The same terms I'll tell you to give, in Chapter 20.

On several occasions I've had physicians who are still in training ask me if there are such things as employment agencies that recruit physicians for industry, government, group practices,

*(Continued on page 16)*

FIGURE 1-5 ═══════════════════════════════════════

## Questions to Ask Before

The group needs to know about you, but you need to know about it if you're to put your professional future in its hands. The questions that follow were developed by the American Group Practice Association with the help of the American Medical Association and the Medical Group Practice Association. They're reprinted here with permission.

### Group History and Philosophy

1. Why was this group started? What has been and is its principal motivation and purpose?
2. What has been the turnover of members? Why have members left the group?
3. What are the professional requirements to become a full-time associate?
4. How long must one be associated with the group to become a full member?
5. How much daily direct supervision will you have from senior members in professional matters? Are you comfortable with this arrangement?
6. Is free and easy consultation among the group physicians a real and actual fact?
7. Do you feel you will be compatible with prospective associates?
8. What degree of harmony exists within the group? What conflicts have had to be resolved?
9. If a multispecialty group, what is the balance of specialties represented? What are the plans to broaden the range of specialties?
10. What are the policies of the group for professional advancement not only in organized medicine but in the academic areas; also, what are the attitudes toward planning group education programs and available time for continuing medical education?
11. What are the future plans of the group, both philosophical and physical?
12. What is the group's policy regarding referral of patients back to local physicians who have referred them to group members?
13. Does the group rate well with local physicians in matters of referral and consultation?
14. What are the policies of the group regarding regular medical conferences?
15. What are the group's policies or requirements concerning mandatory and voluntary retirement?
16. What is the legal structure of the group—partnership, professional association, professional corporation?
17. What is your initial rapport with members of the group?
18. What will be your approximate patient load?

## Accepting a Group's Offer

### Community Relations

1. What is the reputation of this group in its community?
2. What is the drawing area for patients?
3. What are the group's relations with the local medical profession?
4. How is this group located with reference to local hospital facilities?
5. Does group membership enhance or hamper a physician in gaining privileges and status in the local hospital?
6. What are the local facilities for a satisfying social and cultural life?

### Finances and Physical Properties

1. Can you reach full equity?
2. What initial investment is required?
3. What further investment is required on becoming a member?
4. How is income distributed among members of the group?
5. Does board certification entitle one to a larger share of net income?
6. What is the financial stability of the group?
7. What are the economic benefits?
   a. Vacations, time off for study, meetings, etc.?
   b. Sick leave, hospitalization, and medical insurance?
   c. Retirement pension?
   d. Practice costs, operation of car?
   e. Dues of professional societies?
   f. Life, malpractice, and other insurance?
8. What general policies govern the setting of fees?
9. How much may one expect to earn after 5 years? After 10 years?
10. Are the diagnostic and technical facilities adequate?
11. What are the possibilities for expansion of the physical plant?
12. Are parking facilities adequate?
13. Is the management considered able and efficient?
14. Are the physicians free of management problems?
15. Is there a minimum guaranteed salary? If so, how can you exceed it?
16. How much of overhead percentage is physicians' benefits, and how much is just cost of doing business?

and other places. Yes, there certainly are. The chances are good that you'll find their ads in your Sunday newspaper. Look, too, for ads placed by the organizations themselves. In this chapter I quote from ads that appeared in Sunday editions of The New York Times, which carries, in its Week in Review section, several pages of display advertising under the heading "Health Care/Hospital/ Medical Employment Opportunities." The major metropolitan newspaper in the part of the country where you want to work may very well have the same kind of advertising section, so it can't hurt to look for it in the Sunday edition.

Also, you can check the Journal of the American Medical Association and the telephone directory's Yellow Pages for employment agencies that serve physicians. Examples of such agencies: Saffer, 505 Fifth Ave., New York 10017; World Wide Health Consultants, Inc., 1271 Avenue of the Americas, New York 10020; Dorothea Bowlby Medical Employment Bureau, 8 South Michigan Ave., Chicago 60603; Technical Personnel, 880 TenMain Center, Kansas City, Mo. 64105; HSRI, 715 East 3900 South (Suite 205), Salt Lake City 84107; and Blendow, Crowley & Oliver, Inc., 420 Lexington Ave., New York 10017.

And don't overlook the American Medical Association, 535 North Dearborn St., Chicago 60610. It maintains a placement office for both permanent and short-term opportunities of all kinds.

If you're the least bit interested in working for government, then don't overlook the professional placement division of your state's employment service. You'll probably find a number of employment opportunities listed there for physicians in a wide variety of assignments in Federal, state, and local governments.

As for compensation, you'll need to compare any salaried offer with the money you'd make in private practice. You may be able to anticipate the production of $60,000 in your first year, depending on all kinds of factors—including the need for your services where you practice, your willingness to keep your nose to the grindstone, your ability, how well organized you are, and your particular specialty.

Remember, though, production is merely the value of your services, not the money actually collected. If you produce $60,000, you'll be lucky to collect $50,000—not necessarily because of inefficiencies in your office or ignorance of practice management, but because you can expect other doctors in the community to dump their deadbeats on you. By the time you end up paying the rent, the help, and the other bills, you may net about $25,000.

Bad? Considering your potential, not so bad. But no question about it: Your financial potential for the first year is better elsewhere. It's not hard to find salaries or guarantees from group practices of $25,000 for the first year.

Longer-range, it's hard to find a job that offers anything approaching the financial potential of private practice. And I'm not just talking about how much you may clear yearly once you're reasonably well established as a practitioner. That will amount to $80,000—or much more if you're above average in managing your time, your career, and your practice. In addition, as Figure 1-2 shows, the right retirement plan can mean a nest egg of well over a million, even at bank interest, if you start soon enough. That's the pot at the end of the private-practice rainbow. And it's well within your grasp because you'll be making the decisions; you won't be trapped in situations created by the bad decisions of others.

# 2

# Going it alone:
# Not so scary, considering
# these sources of help

You're anxious to know how much it will cost you to repay a start-up loan and where you can get it. O.K. Let's get right to it.

You've always got to estimate your financial future for purposes of budgeting. That's basic management. For your purposes, figure on first-year production—the value of fees for services you'll render—at $60,000. Now, it's tough to set aside an amount equal to 6 to 9 per cent of production for debt service, but that's just about what you need to do to get started right, unless you can find better terms than those you're *likely* to encounter.

What you can expect is a loan from a commercial bank with an interest rate in the neighborhood of 12 per cent. The payments for, say, $15,000 worth of leasehold improvements, fixtures, furnishings, and equipment will run about $330 monthly for five years; for $20,000 worth, about $440. Each $50 of monthly payment represents an amount equal to 1 per cent of your projected first-year production.

## Getting started in private practice

When you go out shopping for a loan, don't be put off if the first responses are negative. They very well may be, too, since bankers are not known to be among our more creative citizens. Many of them, as you'd suspect, aren't about to lend money to anyone unless he's so wealthy that he doesn't really need the loan. Doctors right out of training usually have little or no collateral, and to many a banker it's unbelievable that anyone thinking of starting a practice would have the audacity to approach his bank for a loan without collateral more than sufficient to cover the amount of the funds he seeks.

Fortunately, not all bankers think that way. You may need to approach every bank listed in the Yellow Pages, but the chances are good that, if you do, you'll find a friendly, creative loan officer who is, if not exactly eager, somewhat predisposed to take a chance on you. New York's Manufacturers Hanover Trust Co., for instance, has a doctor plan in its small-business loan department. It's open to physicians who have not yet entered practice and who have no financial track record to speak of. That doesn't mean Manufacturers Hanover will hand money over to just any turkey who skips into one of its offices. You have to go to the personal loan department of any branch and talk with a loan officer there. The interview is extremely important. The loan officer has got to get the impression that you're a responsible, serious-minded person who's adequately trained for private practice, suited to it by temperament, and, of course, trustworthy, loyal, helpful, friendly, cour-

FIGURE 2-1 ═══════════════════════════════════════

### Monthly Payments for Five-Year Start-Up Loan

| Borrowed | 9% | 9½% | 10% | 11% | 12% | 14% | 15% |
|---|---|---|---|---|---|---|---|
| | | | Rate of Interest | | | | |
| $ 1,000 | $ 20.76 | $ 21.01 | $ 21.25 | $ 21.75 | $ 22.25 | $ 23.27 | $ 23.79 |
| 15,000 | 311.38 | 315.03 | 318.71 | 326.14 | 333.67 | 349.03 | 356.85 |
| 20,000 | 415.17 | 420.04 | 424.95 | 434.85 | 444.89 | 465.37 | 475.80 |

Reprinted with permission from *The Thorndike Encyclopedia of Banking and Financial Tables. 1978 Yearbook.* Copyright 1977 Warren Gorham & Lamont Inc., 210 South Street, Boston, Mass. 02111.

## THE EDGEWATER HOSPITAL
### SATELLITE BUDGET

|  | FIRST YEAR |
|---|---|
| **Expense:** | |
| Personnel | |
| RN - Nurse P.T. | $ 50,000 |
| Lab. Tech F.T. | 18,000 |
| Clerk-Typist F.T. | 14,000 |
| Fringe Benefits | 9,000 |
|  | 34,750 |
| Total - Personnel | $125,750 |
| | |
| **Other:** | |
| General Liability Insurance | $ 2,500 |
| Utilities | 2,000 |
| Telephone | 1,500 |
| Water & sewer | 500 |
| Medical Supplies | 2,500 |
| Janitor Service | 1,500 |
| Scavenger | 1,000 |
| Contingency | 6,500 |
| Total - Facility Service | $ 18,000 |
| | |
| Rent | $ 15,000 |
| Office Renovation | |

Capital Items*

| | |
|---|---|
| Furniture | $ 10,000 |
| Centrifuge | 500 |
| Microscope | 1,650 |
| Otoscope & Ophthalmoscope (in carrying case) 2 @$200 ea. | 400 |
| Blood Pressure Kit (Wall Mounted) 2 @$100 ea. | 200 |
| EKG Machine | 1,500 |
| | $ 14,250 |

*Furniture & equipment may be procured for book value at any time by the physician.

teous, kind, obedient, cheerful, thrifty, brave, clean, and reverent.

Loan rates are subject to change with the weather, but Manufacturers Hanover was recently charging 9.58 per cent on small-business loans repayable in 12 months and 11.96 per cent when repayable in five years. Obviously, this bank wants to see its loans repaid in five years; you should be prepared to pay maximum, and something on the order of 12 per cent.

On the West Coast, in the Midwest, in the South, and in other places in between, you'll find a reception approximately equal in warmth at an occasional bank. For instance, at Wells Fargo Bank, which has 330 branches throughout California, a loan officer will go out of his way to figure out a reason to grant you the loan you need for start-up funds, or so I'm told by the bank's public relations department.

The competing Bank of America has the same attitude. According to its public relations department, that bank stands ready to offer new physicians amounts ranging from $20,000 to $50,000 toward the purchase of clinical equipment, reception-room furniture, fixtures, furnishings, and the like. Bank of America also has an equipment-leasing program that provides a line of credit up to $15,000. The bank has 1,088 branches throughout California, and in those located near medical buildings you'll find specialists in handling loan discussions with doctors.

A third California example is Security Pacific National Bank, which has what it calls a doctor-dentist assistance plan. The plan consists of three segments: life-insurance premium financing, equipment financing and working capital loans, and a revolving line of credit. How do you get in on the plan? A vice president of the bank told me, "It's most essential that the lending officer be satisfied by recommendation that the new doctor has every chance of success in the profession."

When I suggest that you approach all the banks listed in the Yellow Pages, I don't mean that you should do so by wearing out your shoe leather. Instead, take the easy way out, and compose a short letter, asking if the bank has any special loan program or consideration for physicians just getting started in practice. Send a copy of the letter to each bank. You could even include photocopies of the first few pages of this chapter; a banker who's never given much thought to a plan for new doctors might do so in response to what he reads here.

You can send the letter to a few savings and loan associations and savings banks, but the response there is less likely to be positive. That's not because savings institutions employ duller people than commercial banks, but because they have restrictions on the kinds of loans they can make. As of early 1978, a mutual savings bank in my state, New Jersey, could lend no more than $5,500 on an unsecured personal loan, with a maximum repayment term of three years. Commercial banks, savings bank officers admit, offer far more flexible terms. Still, don't give up the idea of finding start-up capital at savings institutions. They've been successfully pushing in recent years for greater latitude in the kinds of business they do, and they're making inroads into areas once considered the exclusive domain of the commercial banks.

As long as you're sending letters out, consider checking the Yellow Pages for the names and addresses of companies in the equipment-leasing business. Understand, now, that there are two kinds of equipment leases—financial and operating. The financial kind is generally offered by a financial institution, the operating kind by a company that actually sells and services the equipment. What I'm suggesting here is that you check with the financial kind.

Do so before you even go out and look at any equipment—

FIGURE 2-2 ═══════════════════════════════════════════

## How Florida Helps

"The Florida Medical Association placement service publishes the Medical Opportunities Bulletin, which outlines all the available opportunities currently listed. The bulletin also provides information on licensing and on how to advertise in the Florida Medical Association Journal, a map of Florida showing the various county locations, the names and addresses of specialty-society secretaries, and the addresses and phone numbers of county medical societies. I'm the contact person for physicians who are interested in locating in Florida."—Robert J. Harvey, Director, Medical Services Department, Florida Medical Association, P.O. Box 2411, 735 Riverside Ave., Jacksonville 32203.

quite possibly, even before you've left training. The idea is to line up your sources of financing as early in the game as possible; that's the step that precedes the selection of equipment. When dealing with either a bank or a leasing company—and remember, some banks offer leasing plans, too—you'll be told the maximum amount of money you can spend. *Then* you can go out and select your equipment.

You'll get all the details of the equipment lease from the lending officer, but what it comes down to is this: You make all the arrangements for the delivery of the equipment, and the financial institution pays for it. Later, you repay the financial institution on the terms you discussed. But make no mistake about it: The equipment is yours, whether it's in your office on purchase or there on a financial lease.

One leasing company that has taken the trouble to point out that it's eager to do business with new physicians is the Hertz Corporation. Its national sales manager for commercial leasing, Alan Quinn, is the man who oversees loans to new practitioners. As I write these words, he's located at the Hertz home offices, 660 Madison Ave., New York 10021. "Yes," he tells me, "we look very favorably on applications from doctors."

You may find that other leasing firms listed in your telephone directory's Yellow Pages take an equally warm attitude toward you, but, again, don't be put off if the initial reaction is negative. In the financing business, no one firm speaks for another. If you look hard enough, you can usually find capital to get a good, small business going. Sooner or later, it's bound to occur to lots more loan officers that physicians in private practice are very good risks.

Chances are that you'll need to get your seed money from such a financial institution or from your family or friends. The best way for a relative or friend to help you out is to lend you his credit, rather than his money, by cosigning your loan or lease. By so doing, he promises to pay if you default. He, like you, may be asked to fill out a loan application and a financial statement, but, as long as you make the loan payments, your relative or friend will pay nothing. It's almost the same thing as his making the loan to you, except that the arrangement is more businesslike.

## Getting started in private practice

You can also get help from a small community that's looking to recruit a doctor. A pair of internists, Dr. Douglas Turtzo and Dr. Peter Ghatak, started up not so long ago with the help of the citizens of Wind Gap, Pa., in an old, unused school building. The town council made the building available for $100 a month during their first four years in practice. They could have found even more attractive terms at any number of other rural communities.

You can even arrange to be paid while you look over a place that may be eager to recruit you. Just take a $500-a-week, short-term assignment in Project U.S.A., the American Medical Association's program that recruits physicians for service in communities that need them. The openings are advertised from time to time in American Medical News, an A.M.A. publication. You can write for information about the program to John Naughton, American Medical Association, 535 North Dearborn St., Chicago 60610.

The A.M.A.'s department of practice management (at the same address) can also give you some help. For instance, it can send you, for only $10, its New Doctor's Kit (Order No. OP458), which contains the following publications: "Planning Guide for Physicians' Medical Facilities," "The Business Side of Medical Practice," "Group Practice Guidelines," "Preparing a Patient Information Booklet," and "Talking With Patients." The kit also

FIGURE 2-3 ════════════════════════════════════════

### How Oregon Helps

"The Oregon Medical Association has a luncheon get-together that coincides with the quarterly meeting of the state's Board of Medical Examiners. We invite each exam-taking doctor and spouse to a Saturday social hour and buffet luncheon. We also invite our own staff and officers, physicians, hospital and community representatives, and others who are trying to recruit doctors. We've found that the luncheon provides an excellent opportunity to introduce the new doctors to the benefits of membership in the society and for them to get acquainted with some practitioners with experience in the state. Several doctors have found permanent places in practice as a direct result of the contacts made."—Ms. Lee Lewis, Director, Physician Placement Service, Oregon Medical Association, 5210 S.W. Corbett Ave., Portland, Ore. 97201.

contains an order form for "Current Procedural Terminology" and a uniform health-insurance claim form, medicolegal forms, and information on A.M.A. membership and placement services. It's a nice, inexpensive package, the brainstorm of my old friend Maynard Heacox, who runs the department and is always on the lookout for new ways for the A.M.A. to be of service to new practitioners.

You'll find that the state medical societies offer lots of help, too. For example, the California Medical Association, 731 Market St., San Francisco 94103, runs a two-day practice management workshop entitled, "Establishing Yourself in Medical Practice." The program covers these topics: personnel problems, patient-flow techniques, physical aspects of the medical office, paperwork (both clinical and financial), practice location, relationships with hospitals and colleagues and the community, pensions, taxes, professional corporations, and medicolegal considerations.

The California Medical Association also publishes a periodic physician-placement bulletin which shows employment and private-practice opportunities of every conceivable description. It also includes the addresses and phone numbers of all the county societies in the state.

State societies elsewhere offer the same kinds of services. The Kentucky Medical Association, for instance, sponsors a three-day seminar that's designed to assist new physicians in establishing their practices. It also provides a physician-placement service—a continuing dialogue between employers looking for doctor-employees, senior physicians searching for young colleagues, and young doctors seeking out opportunities for solo practice.

Local county societies often offer new practitioners a great deal of help, too. The St. Louis Medical Society, for instance, has a classified section in its twice-monthly publication that lists opportunities of interest to doctors looking for employment, a partner or group to join, or a practice to buy. In addition, the St. Louis Medical Society has a no-fee employment agency to help practitioners staff their offices with medical assistants; 10 different group insurance policies, including health, disability, life, and office liability coverages; practice management seminars, including medical student forums; a telephone answering service that's owned in part by the society; a 55,000-volume medical library; and both scientific and management educational programs, which are conducted in the society's own 750-seat auditorium and 250-seat banquet room.

Many local societies—county societies, for the most part, but also some that serve more than one county or a specific major city—offer outstanding continuing-education programs for their members. For example, the Berks County Medical Society in Pennsylvania runs a two-hour accredited course from 9:30 to 11:30 the first three Wednesday mornings of each month. And, like so many other county societies, it offers society-endorsed group insurance and a prototype retirement plan for self-employed and incorporated physicians.

In New Jersey's Bergen County, my own home county, executive director George Willis maintains a list, by specialty and by location, of medical offices throughout the county. He makes a point of knowing which communities and hospitals need specific specialists, and so he, like many other paid directors of county societies, is a good person to consult about a likely location to open a practice.

And, like the A.M.A., Willis provides a kit for new practitioners. The kit includes a checklist of steps you *must* take (such as register your license to practice at the County Clerk's office); *should* take (apply for malpractice insurance); and will probably *want* to take (inquire about a telephone answering service). The kit also includes the phone numbers of the agent who sells the society-endorsed malpractice coverage, the county's hospitals, and key community health resources agencies, such as Visiting Nurses and the Poison Control Center.

Some county societies offer specific office-support services— a telephone answering service, say; or, as in the case of Ohio's Montgomery County Medical Society, a centralized billing service and a full time collection agency. The Montgomery County Medical Society also runs a community blood center that serves its own county and some surrounding counties.

Both state and local societies are good sources of information about part-time employment opportunities through which new

**26**

practitioners can supplement their incomes—Government institutions, industry, state and county hospitals, schools, labor unions, and insurance examinations.

Local societies and sometimes hospital administrators, too, can help a new solo practitioner get coverage for his off-hours. They can help him join an established coverage group or launch a new one. Successful examples are often composed of no more than five or six doctors whose practices are geographically nearby, in the same specialty, and serving the same hospital. Coverage groups of more than five or six physicians tend to break up after repeated disagreements.

When it comes to getting hospital appointments, you can run into an impossible problem. In big cities, it's a rare general practitioner who's allowed inside the door of a voluntary hospital. But just the opposite situation often exists in small-town hospitals, where specialists tend to be shunned by the G.P.s who control appointments. In suburban areas where hospital expansion hasn't kept pace with population growth, *any* new doctor can have a hard time getting in.

Court decisions have established that no one has a right to hospital privileges simply because he's a licensed physician. He must qualify for staff membership under the institution's bylaws; at a minimum, they require him to be a graduate of a recognized school, to have a state license, and to conform with other state laws governing medical practice.

In many places, a tax-supported hospital must allow at least courtesy privileges to all local applicants who measure up to its standards. But a voluntary hospital can be more discriminating—requiring, if it wishes, board certification or a university teaching appointment. A proprietary hospital makes its own rules; some welcome any doctor who will help fill its beds, but others accept only physician-stockholders.

So you don't dare decide on a location without getting some encouragement from either a hospital administrator or a chief of service. Before you inquire about available office space, check out the hospital situation.

*(Continued on page 30)*

FIGURE 2-4 ═══════════════════════════════════════════════════

## Addresses of State Placement Offices

☐ Medical Association of the State of Alabama, 19 South Jackson St., Montgomery 36104.

☐ Alaska State Medical Association, 1135 West Eighth Ave., Anchorage 99501.

☐ Arizona Medical Association, Inc., 810 West Bethany Home Rd., Phoenix 85013.

☐ Arkansas Medical Society, 214 North 12th, P.O. Box 1208, Fort Smith 72901.

☐ California Medical Association, 731 Market St., San Francisco 94103.

☐ Colorado Medical Society, 1601 East 19th Ave., Denver 80218.

☐ Connecticut State Medical Society, 160 St. Ronan St., New Haven 06511.

☐ Medical Society of Delaware, 1925 Lovering Ave., Wilmington 19806.

☐ Medical Society of the District of Columbia, 2007 Eye St., N.W., Washington, D.C. 20006.

☐ Florida Medical Association, P.O. Box 2411, Jacksonville 32203.

☐ Medical Association of Georgia, 938 Peachtree St., N.E., Atlanta 30309.

☐ Hawaii Medical Association, 510 South Beretania St., Honolulu 96813.

☐ Idaho Medical Association, 407 West Bannock St., Boise 83702.

☐ Illinois State Medical Society, 360 North Michigan Ave., Chicago 60601.

☐ Indiana State Medical Association, 3935 North Meridian, Indianapolis 46208.

☐ Iowa Medical Society, 1001 Grand Ave., West Des Moines 50265.

☐ Kansas Medical Society, 1300 Topeka Blvd., Topeka 66612.

☐ Kentucky Medical Association, 3532 Ephraim McDowell Dr., Louisville 40205.

☐ Louisiana State Medical Society, 1700 Josephine St., New Orleans 70113.

☐ Maine Medical Association, P.O. Box 250, Brunswick 04011.

☐ Medical and Chirurgical Faculty of Maryland, 1211 Cathedral St., Baltimore 21201.

☐ Massachusetts Medical Society, 22 The Fenway, Boston 02215.

☐ Michigan Health Council, 712 Abbott Rd., P.O. Box 1010, East Lansing 48823.

☐ Minnesota State Medical Association, 375 Jackson St., St. Paul 55101.

☐ Mississippi State Medical Association, 735 Riverside Dr., P.O. Box 5207, Jackson 39216.

☐ Missouri State Medical Association, 515 East High St., P.O. Box 1028, Jefferson City 65101.

☐ Montana Medical Association, 2021 11th Ave., Helena 59601.

☐ Nebraska Medical Association, 1902 First National Bank Bldg., Lincoln 68508.

☐ Nevada State Medical Association, 3660 Baker Lane, Reno 89502.

☐ New Hampshire Medical Society, 4 Park St., Concord 03301.

☐ Medical Society of New Jersey, P.O. Box 904, 315 West State St., Trenton 08605.

☐ New Mexico Medical Society, 3010 Monte Vista Blvd., N.E., Albuquerque 87106.

☐ Medical Society of the State of New York, 420 Lakeville Rd., Lake Success 11040.

☐ North Carolina Medical Society, P.O. Box 27167, 222 North Person St., Raleigh 27611.

☐ North Dakota Medical Association, M.D.U. Office Bldg., Suite 307, Box 1198, Bismarck 58501.

☐ Ohio State Medical Association, 17 South High St., Suite 500, Columbus 43215.

☐ Oklahoma State Medical Association, 601 N.W. Expressway, Oklahoma City 73118.

☐ Oregon Medical Association, 5210 S.W. Corbett Ave., Portland 97201.

☐ Pennsylvania Medical Society, 20 Erford Rd., Lemoyne 17043.

☐ Rhode Island Medical Society, 106 Francis St., Providence 02903.

☐ South Carolina Medical Association, 1508 Washington St., Suite 201, Box 11188, Columbia 29211.

☐ South Dakota State Medical Association, 711 North Lake Ave., Sioux Falls 57104.

☐ Tennessee Medical Association, 112 Louise Ave., Nashvillle 37203.

☐ Texas Medical Association, 1801 North Lamar Blvd., Austin 78701.

☐ Utah State Medical Association, 42 South Fifth East St., Salt Lake City 84102.

☐ Vermont State Medical Society, 128 Merchants Row, Rutland 05701.

☐ Virginia Council on Health and Medical Care, 100 East Franklin St., Richmond 23219.

☐ Washington State Medical Association, 444 Northeast Ravenna Blvd., Seattle 98115.

☐ West Virginia State Medical Association, 1526 Charleston National Plaza, Box 1031, Charleston 25324.

☐ State Medical Society of Wisconsin, 330 East Lakeside, Box 1109, Madison 53701.

☐ Wyoming State Medical Society, 412 Randall Ave., P.O. Box 1387, Cheyenne 82001.

Source: American Medical Association.

## Getting started in private practice

That's high on the agenda of those management consultants who go out of their way to provide services to new practitioners. Robert C. Fraim is such an example. I've long known him to be among that group of consultants, so I wrote to him not long ago and asked just how far he's prepared to go for a client soon to enter practice, and he replied:

"When asked by a young man or woman still in training, I'll put him in practice anywhere in the United States he wants to go—with absolutely no participation on his part except to identify the community in which he wishes to practice. I'll go to that city, select an office, remodel it if necessary, acquire his equipment, hire his people, develop his appointment system, send out his announcement cards, and do everything else that's necessary so that, when he finishes his training the latter part of June, we'll meet at his new office, and I'll introduce him to his new employees, walk him through the office, and introduce him to his first patient."

That's marvelous service, and now that Fraim has let the world know about it, I'm sure any number of other management consultants will be following his lead. Of course, many of the management men and women have long provided less comprehensive assistance. Some examples: "Evaluating an offer from a group or an individual physician" (Donald L. Anderholz). "Obtaining proper financing, planning office efficiency, selecting office equipment, hiring office personnel, collecting fees, and acquiring new patients" (E.A. Thieman). "Helping a new doctor buy an established practice or go into such a practice with a senior physician on fair terms" (Melvin L. Schultz).

Fees for such services vary. Some consultants work for new doctors on a reduced-fee basis. "We charge half the regular fee for the first six months of continuing service" (Charles H. Walsh).

Scaring up the necessary bread may be the least of your troubles in going solo. In fact, you may be better off than getting hooked up with established practitioners unwilling to offer fair terms. The help that's available to a solo practitioner is substantial, and it can be far more sophisticated than the help you get from older doctors. Chapter 20 deals with buying into a practice.

# Beware the jackals: They may get you before you're out of training

That's when they got Florida family practitioner, Fred Bodner. While he was still in training, an insurance guy buddied up to him, did him favors, even lent him money.

Oh, boy, did he ever!

I first met Dr. Bodner after he'd been in practice about three years. That's when he called me in to see if I could help him figure a way out of his financial mess. The man was 32 years old, drove a Mercedes even then, regularly vacationed out of the country, skied at Vail two weeks every winter, and lived in the most expensive house in his neighborhood. But his financial troubles started back when he first started borrowing money from his insurance buddy. Now he owed the guy more than $12,000 for life-insurance premiums he'd paid on the doctor's behalf. "Do I have to pay? How can I get out of this debt?" my new client asked.

Well, he had signed papers acknowledging the debt, so I told him that, though it was a good idea to check the point with a friendly lawyer, he'd better plan on paying up—either by floating a bank loan or by making arrangements with the insurance man to pay off the debt in reasonable installments.

I know of many other instances in which doctors have gotten themselves into financial hot water. Like Dr. Bodner, many seem to have jumped in with an early purchase of life insurance. Even so, I do *not* think that many insurance salespersons are deliberately underhanded. Rather, their training is such that they tend to believe in what they sell—all logic to the contrary.

When I talk about insurance-sales training, I don't speak lightly. About 10 years ago I went undercover, you might say. I underwent training as a life-insurance salesman, passed the state licensing examination (and, while I was at it, the National Association of Securities Dealers exam, too), and actually went out into the field, where I worked for an agency and sold whole-life insurance for a couple of months. I've written about insurance quite a bit since then.

The strange part of this whole insurance thing is that it's a necessary and desirable product. If there weren't life insurance, someone would invent it. For relatively little money (at least at your age), you can assure your wife and children of financial security for the rest of their lives.

For example, $300,000 of straight term protection may cost you roughly $735 at age 30. If your wife puts that $300,000 in a savings bank, she can get more than $24,000 a year.

But I'll bet you a dollar that you've never heard such figures from any insurance man. Those who chase doctors in training are almost never selling yearly renewable term insurance, what many people call pure insurance. Those salesmen are sometimes selling endowment life-insurance coverage, but more often they're selling *whole*-life insurance, which also goes by the terms ordinary life and permanent life. Different salesmen use different terms, but all three terms mean exactly the same thing.

They sell a lot of that kind of coverage for three reasons: Mostly, they wear people down until they buy or, in a version of that approach, get buddy-buddy with their prey, as in the case of Dr. Bodner; they offer the lure of something for nothing; and they offer this terrific money-saving deal that's called *minimum deposit.*

Well, if there's any such thing as something for nothing, you won't find it in the life-insurance industry. The cash value or savings feature found in endowment, whole-life, and other cash-value coverages amounts to America's single biggest consumer fraud, as has been authoritatively described in Congressional testimony. The minimum deposit ploy compounds the felony.

To get some idea of the financial implications, look at that $735 a 30-year-old might pay for $300,000 of pure insurance. To get a bigger commission bite out of the $735, a salesman will try to sell some kind of cash-value coverage, which, depending on the company and the specific policy, may provide not $300,000 of protection but only a third as much, or even less. So young family heads, who can afford to spend no more than, say, $735 for life-insurance protection, settle for $40,000 to $100,000 of coverage, instead of the full $300,000.

Chances are that they buy the cash-value coverage in the expectation of getting something for nothing. They expect to get their money back. Cash-value coverage is, as your friendly insurance salesman may have told you, a combination of insurance and a savings account.

What he probably hasn't told you is that your dollars would buy much more protection with yearly renewable term insurance; that the cash-value insurance won't pay your family a nickel more if you die, despite the addition of the savings factor; that, if you live to cash in the savings portion of the policy when you're old, the money you get back will be far less than the money you'd paid in (unless, maybe, you wait until you're almost 100 years old before cashing it in); that the purchasing power of money you do get back will be so severely eroded by inflation that it will be worth far, far less than the premium dollars you'd paid in; and that you'd have done far better by putting the difference between the premium for yearly renewable term and the premium for an equal amount of cash-value coverage in a bank savings account.

If you save that difference, you'll have the full amount of protection from the yearly renewable term insurance *plus* the bank savings. And if you outlive your need for the coverage, you can quietly drop the insurance. You'll get back nothing for it, to be sure, but your savings account at the bank will contain far more money than you would have gotten back from the cash-value policy.

The argument in favor of minimum deposit is that you can—after four years of paying the full, regular premiums for cash-value insurance—pay something like the premium for term insurance. What you may not be told is that minimum deposit also reduces the amount of protection.

Unbelievable. But there's more. The amount you pay during those four years may very well be enough to set you up in practice or to buy an X-ray machine or a car. For example, if a whole-life policy costs $11,760 in four years, the price of a term policy over those same years may be only $2,940—a difference of $8,820.

The insurance man's counterargument? "You'd better be careful, Doc, because yearly renewable term insurance increases in price every year!"

Oh, wow! Everybody hates rising prices, right? So it's an effective argument. The trouble with it is that the annual price rise is slight. A typical increase for a $300,000 policy is from $735 at age 30 to $744 at age 31—lots less than the premium you'd pay for whole life at that age—generally, $2,200 to $5,100, depending on the insurer. You may be pushing age 50 before you see the annual premium on a term policy rise to the level of the premium of whole-life at age 30. By then, you'll probably need less life-insurance protection and quite possibly none at all if your Keogh or professional-corporation retirement plan goes as well as it should—even assuming that you go for no more of a return than savings-bank interest. And if you put the difference in premiums for the two kinds of policies in a savings bank, from age 30 through 55 you'll have put more than $14,600 there—and that the *minimum* difference between premiums over those years.

The next sad finding I have to report is that, despite all I've said here and despite any reinforcing facts and opinions you may get from other management consultants or financial advisers, you'll still buy the cash-value policy. At least, you will if you're typical. Insurance companies don't invest piles of money in training their salesmen for nothing. Any of the next 10 insurance guys you meet will be more than pleased to pick apart everything I've said here—and they can do it, because there's not an argument, no matter how sound, that people peddling cash-value policies aren't trained to counter. But if you're foolish enough to rely on the advice of salesmen whose livelihoods depend on your buying what they're selling, then perhaps you'd better seek out the arguments of salesmen who sell only the yearly renewable term coverage.

You'll probably have to go looking for someone like that. His commission on each sale is small, so he tries to cut his sales expenses by asking clients to see him at his office, and he tends to deal with relatively sophisticated purchasers. In Chapter 21 you'll find a list of some of the companies that specialize in yearly renewable term insurance (Figure 21-2). You can find a nearby term specialist by writing to the home office of one of those companies.

My comment about how salesmen earn their money points up the way to tell the difference between a salesman and a consultant. Though it's true that some salesmen are on straight salary, most earn their money by getting commissions on what they sell. A true consultant, however, is paid for his expertise and his objectivity. He gets paid for telling you what to buy, whether you accept his advice or not.

A consultant who takes a commission on your purchase of insurance or other goods or services is not a true consultant at all but a salesman who calls himself a consultant. That's going to be important for you to remember, because there are a growing number of such salesmen.

Many of your older colleagues have incorporated their practices through the services of such people, who use the setting up of a professional corporation as a wedge to get through the door and to sell lots of life, disability, and health insurance to the doctors and their medical assistants. The convincing feature is the old something-for-nothing bit. The doctors' retirement plans and other fringe-benefit plans are prepared for free or for a reduced price.

Of course, there's nothing free about the arrangement at all. Life insurance in a retirement plan means that retirement-plan dollars are put into insurance rather than into compounded tax-free earnings. The difference is anything but free service.

## Getting started in private practice

As we've seen, $2,200 can buy a whole-life policy or it can earn 8 per cent interest in a savings bank and do so tax-free if it's in a retirement plan. Over 25 years, that amount compounds in the bank to a total of more than $180,700. That's a big savings account to give up just for the privilege of saving a few hundred dollars in professional-corporation start-up expenses.

That's not to say that *all* salesmen-consultants are to be avoided like highwaymen. Though everyone I've ever known in the insurance field is really a salesman, no matter how else he represents himself, some persons in other fields—interior decoration, office-equipment consulting, and real-estate consulting, for instance—truly are consultants but work for a fee expressed as some percentage of the cost of what's purchased or on some other fee basis. In such cases there's no magic way to tell the difference between salesmen and consultants. You've got to rely on the reputation of the person.

Don't be taken in by the fact that some consultants are licensed by the state. Such licensing can be misleading. People often assume that, because someone is licensed, he's also endorsed and presumably competent. Well, that's not a law of nature.

States license insurance salesmen, certified public accountants, lawyers, and some others, including physicians, but the state licensing may only be evidence that the person has paid a fee. Not all licensed professionals need to show evidence of competence. In New Jersey, passing my insurance licensing exam proved only that I had absorbed a certain amount of my employer's training. And my National Association of Securities Dealers exam didn't prove much more, but it brought me the legal right to sell mutual funds and certain other investments.

People who sell investments go by different names—stockbrokers, customers' men, account executives—and most of them are licensed, but make no mistake about it: They're salesmen, not consultants. Now and then you'll hear of one who takes the long view and puts his clients' needs first. But that kind is a rarity. Most investment salesmen take the short view; they're interested only in closing the immediate sale. In their marketplace any argument leading to a closing is good and proper unless it's clearly *illegal*.

36

Since licensing means little, it shouldn't bother you that there are few or no licensing requirements by any state or other public body for estate planners, personal financial managers, business managers, retirement advisers, financial advisers, tax advisers, or management consultants.

Most of the people who call themselves estate planners are really insurance salesmen. So are some personal financial managers, business advisers, retirement advisers, and financial advisers— all terms in common use. The fact that any one of them will take the commission on an insurance sale doesn't necessarily mean that he isn't truly expert at what he does or that he puts his own financial interests ahead of his clients' or is to be avoided. Not at all. I'm sure that many such advisers do excellent work on a thoroughly professional level. But as a client or potential client, you need to know the source or sources of your adviser's earnings. Ask him if he minds discussing the matter. Regardless of his income sources, you may be convinced that he's both knowledgeable and honest.

I have somewhat more negative feelings about tax advice. Many people, including a lot of doctors, rely on accountants for tax advice. I know from observation and experience that many of these people are not well served—and for a good reason. Tax advice is based on the interpretation of laws passed by a legislative body and interpreted by the courts. People trained to interpret law and court decisions are called lawyers, not accountants.

Accountants are trained to check the work of bookkeepers— that is, to audit books. That's all. For that reason, I've long been amazed at the way your older colleagues almost universally put blind faith in their accountants' ability to function in the lawyer's domain and, for that matter, to advise them on every conceivable matter directly or indirectly related to dollar investments, putting up buildings, evaluating business deals, whatever.

In fact, many doctors going into practice retain an accountant right off the bat. He may be some guy with an office next door, or, more often, he comes on the recommendation of some older colleague who may or may not know what he's talking about. And the reason the new doctor hires himself an accountant, often even before his office phone is installed, is because he doesn't know

**37**

enough to go down to the Internal Revenue Service office himself and file a Form SS-4, the application for an employer identification number. Believe me, you don't need to put an accountant on retainer to handle your payroll or to fill out a Form SS-4.

Now, I'm *not* saying that accountants never make good tax or financial advisers. Some get enough additional training and practical experience to become truly superior consultants. But these are people who have gone well beyond their basic accounting training. They can do more than check the bookkeeping for accuracy and ledger cards for posting; they do more than fill in the blanks on an income tax form. In fact, many of this country's medical management consultants are accountants who have long specialized in handling the problems of doctor-clients. They call themselves management consultants, rather than accountants, for a very good reason: A great deal of the consulting they do goes well beyond their accounting. There's no way an accountant can deal exclusively with doctor-clients without picking up knowledge of such management-related matters as hiring, firing, training, supervising, staffing, office-space requirements, office equipment, fair terms of partnership, incorporation, and more. With that additional

FIGURE 3-1 ═══════════════════════════════════════

## Some Professional Associations for True Consultants

**Investment consultants**

Investment Counsel Association of America, Inc.
127 East 59th St., New York 10022

**Medical Management Consultants**

Society of Medical-Dental Management Consultants
6100 Golden Valley Rd., Minneapolis 55422

Society of Professional Business Consultants
221 North LaSalle St., Chicago 60601

**Retirement Plan Consultants**

Conference of Actuaries in Public Practice
208 South LaSalle St., Chicago 60604

knowledge, he truly should call himself something more than an accountant.

If he calls himself a medical management consultant or a professional business consultant (many prefer the latter term), he probably belongs to either the Society of Medical-Dental Management Consultants or the Society of Professional Business Consultants. To belong and maintain his membership, a consultant must satisfy either organization's ethics committee that he is a consultant selling expertise and objectivity, not a salesman selling products. Insurance salesmen definitely do not qualify.

However, not all ethical medical management consultants belong to one of those two professional associations. For example, none of the people at Medidentics, Inc., in Park Ridge, Ill., belongs, and that's the largest medical management consulting firm operating under one roof. Also, there's the PM network—a sizable group of ethical consultants, for the most part franchise owners, directed by the Black & Skaggs consulting organization based in Battle Creek, Mich. And there are undoubtedly other ethical, competent organizations and persons who serve physicians well. Just as there's no law stating that a medical management consultant needs to be licensed by the state, there's no law requiring him or her to belong to either of the professional associations.

If I were a physician, I'd feel perfectly comfortable dealing with a member of either society or of the two big independents, Medidentics and PM.

Not necessarily so with lawyers. I've heard many doctors bemoan the quality of their accounting service, but not the way I've heard them complain about their lawyer's level of competence and high fees. Sad to say, the good ones are hard to find. Mind you, I don't expect any professional to work cheap. To gross as much as, say, a physician with a typical well-managed practice, a competent lawyer or other professional must charge more than $635 a day. The high-fee lawyers I'm talking about charge more.

Again, I'm not suggesting that everyone in the field is a bad apple. There are some excellent lawyers around. It's just hard to find them. That's why medical management consultants keep lists of the names and addresses of lawyers who've come highly recommended. That's also the reason why you should look for recommendations on lawyers from colleagues, friends, and family members. You'll need a lawyer to write your will and to revise it whenever there's an addition to your family or some other significant change. You'll need him for the incorporation of your practice or when you take a partner, when you buy your home, and when you enter a business deal.

Far too many professionals who serve doctors put their own interests first by giving advice that's good for the adviser but bad for the doctor. I don't know what the solution to the problem is, but you ought to be aware of it, because you'll probably encounter it. In fact, you'll probably be a victim, sooner or later.

Lawyers, management consultants, and other advisers have learned from dealing with your older colleagues that the adviser who allows a doctor-client to get involved in a business deal or an investment can plan on being fired the moment the deal goes sour. Your colleagues have developed a widespread reputation for asking for advice so that they'll have a scapegoat. On the other hand, not many lawyers or other advisers have ever received a bonus, praise, gratitude, or other acknowledgment for recognizing a good deal and for advising participation. So there's nothing to be gained by urging the doctor-client on.

For the same reason, much tax advice is hopelessly conservative. In fact, it's just plain bad. Your older colleagues have earned a widespread reputation for telling tax advisers to save them every possible penny and for being pleased with the tax savings that result—until the I.R.S. notice of an impending audit arrives in the mail. Some of your colleagues fire their advisers at that moment, apparently not realizing that the only practitioners who are never audited are the ones whose tax returns are prepared and signed by some turkey who's well known in the local I.R.S. auditing division as an adviser who never, but never, gives advice that strays from the tax collector's interpretation. So don't be surprised—or impressed—when you hear an older colleague boast that he's never been audited.

Is that the best route for you to take? Not at all. Though the I.R.S. likes to set itself up as a tax adviser—witness that TV advertising at tax time urging taxpayers to phone the I.R.S. or to drop into the local office for advice on preparing the return—it is, in fact, nothing more than a tax collector. To do its business well, it must collect every dime it can.

The I.R.S. attorneys' interpretations of the law are no more valid than the interpretations of any other reasonably competent lawyer. Or citizen. That's right: If you or any other citizen takes the time and effort and expense to stay current with legislative and judicial tax developments, your interpretations may be every bit as valid, in a Federal court's view, as the I.R.S.'s. Though the I.R.S. has many competent, well-trained, career-minded people on its payroll, it also bears the burden, much to the dismay of those fine people, of many persons of doubtful competence, some of whom are in the I.R.S. only because they know the credit will look good later on a curriculum vitae and help to win them clients or a job.

The recommendations you get from older doctors and friends, even from your family, are not to be accepted unquestioningly, since there's much bad tax advice being sold. But the recommendations need to be sought. You can also stop in at a nearby community, university, or courthouse library and check the Martindale-Hubbell law directory. It shows each lawyer's age, college, law school, specialty, firm affiliation, associates, type of clients, financial standing, and rating by his colleagues for ability. For all that, the directory is not a complete and foolproof guide. But it is, like the recommendations you'll get, a potentially useful step.

Membership in a bar association or in any other legal organization isn't much of a recommendation. The situation is different, though, with two other kinds of advisers—investment advisers and actuaries. Investment advisers belong to a professional organization that bars membership to those who accept sales commissions. Members of the Investment Counsel Association of America, Inc., all claim to be pure investment consultants. And many, though by no means all, members of the Conference of Actuaries in Public Practice are thoroughly independent of insurance sales—an important point, since many actuaries are employed by insurers.

I've told you all this with some misgivings. It's information that you need, but I'd hate to see you become paranoid in your

**41**

dealings with other professionals. There's too much of that among doctors already. In fact, the automatic suspicion and mistrust exhibited by many of your older colleagues is one of the basic reasons so many of them have received bad treatment. If it's hard for you to develop much interest in and to give good service to a patient who clearly mistrusts and dislikes you, then you know what I mean.

Paranoia is by no means the only reason doctors are treated badly. If there's a confidence man in town selling phony cattle or oil deals, snake oil, or any other hustle you can think of, you *know* he'll hit the docs. You need to know why.

The first reason is obvious. Doctors have the money to invest. You're about to become a member of the highest-paid occupational group. Second, there really isn't all that much good advice around. Well, there may be enough of it, but doctors don't always seek it out. One reason: Doctors tend to rely too much on their talent for judging character. Too often, a doctor throws up his hands and gives up trying to unravel the complexities of an insurance plan or an investment deal. Instead, he goes along with the advice given by a financial adviser or salesman because he seems competent and honest.

Face it: The most competent guy in town is the confidence man. He's also the best salesman. The guy who's competent enough to protect your interests and who is highly inclined to do so may not be as handsome or as good a dresser, and he may not be as well spoken or polished, and he may not arrive in as fancy a car. So pay attention to the substance of the advice, not to the style of the adviser.

But perhaps the biggest reason of all why doctors tend to get taken is that so many of them all but ask for what they get. In Chapter 12, you'll find out just what Main Street thinks of your older colleagues, and that view is most likely the biggest burden you have inherited from them.

Consider just the financial situation. A doctor netting six figures is hardly rare; the typical compensation from a well-managed practice in 1977 was more than $85,000, while for *all* practices across the U.S., the typical compensation was more than $58,000—figures that exclude any additional income from investments or earnings by spouses. How are patients doing? Well, the before-tax earnings in the average household stand at less than $15,000. Some resident physicians are paid more than that. Some interns are, too. And in your first year of private practice, the chances are fair to good that you'll be able to net at least twice as much as that.

So be careful, but be kind. Be knowledgeable, too. But that's why you're reading this book, isn't it?

# 4

# How you can find
# the right place to practice

I know you're not going to decide on a place to practice without taking time to talk about hospital privileges, the need for your services, and the community's economic and cultural future. You'll talk with such people as the executive director of the county medical society, the administrators and chiefs of service in your specialty at the leading hospitals, a couple of referring doctors, a banker, and a real-estate agent or two. I also know that you'll take into consideration such factors as the availability of opportunities for your spouse's career, the quality of the schools, recreational facilities in the area and the region, shopping, and, to be sure, climate.

But there's a whole lot of research you need to do before investing the travel time and money to do all that. To begin with, consider the fact that significant population shifts are occurring. Percentages of population growth between 1976 and 1981 will be greatest in the West and Southwest. The Midwest and New England will grow much less.

## Getting started in private practice

Population-movement trends are vital to doctors, because population means patients. Alaska, Arizona, Utah, Nevada, and Florida will show the greatest percentage of population increase from 1976 to 1981. Idaho, Wyoming, New Mexico, Montana, and Colorado will show the next greatest increases. On the other hand, New York may show no change during the period, and five places will lose population—Missouri, New Jersey, Indiana, Pennsylvania, and the District of Columbia.

Population, of course, isn't the full story. If you're going to be

FIGURE 4-1 ══════════════════════════════════════════

### Doctor Opportunity Ratings for the United States

Equal weight is given to the need for doctors and to patients' ability to pay for medical services. U.S.: 100.

| | | | |
|---|---|---|---|
| Alaska | 149 | Maryland | 101 |
| North Dakota | 123 | | |
| South Dakota | 116 | **United States** | **100** |
| Mississippi | 112 | | |
| Iowa | 112 | Minnesota | 100 |
| Arkansas | 111 | Oklahoma | 99 |
| Alabama | 110 | Missouri | 99 |
| South Carolina | 110 | Pennsylvania | 99 |
| Nebraska | 110 | West Virginia | 97 |
| Illinois | 110 | Washington | 97 |
| Indiana | 108 | Hawaii | 97 |
| Wyoming | 108 | New York | 97 |
| North Carolina | 107 | Montana | 96 |
| Kansas | 107 | Michigan | 96 |
| Kentucky | 106 | Massachusetts | 96 |
| Georgia | 105 | New Mexico | 95 |
| Virginia | 105 | Utah | 94 |
| Delaware | 105 | New Hampshire | 94 |
| Nevada | 105 | Rhode Island | 94 |
| Louisiana | 103 | California | 93 |
| Idaho | 103 | Colorado | 92 |
| Texas | 103 | Oregon | 92 |
| Wisconsin | 103 | Maine | 91 |
| Ohio | 103 | Florida | 91 |
| New Jersey | 103 | District of Columbia | 90 |
| Connecticut | 102 | Arizona | 87 |
| Tennessee | 101 | Vermont | 83 |

practical-minded about selecting a location, you also have to consider the ability of patients to pay for medical services.

By 1980, the five most affluent metropolitan areas, measured in terms of effective buying income in a household, will be, in order, Anchorage; the Bridgeport-Stamford-Norwalk-Danbury area of Connecticut; Saginaw, Mich.; Washington, D.C.; and the New Brunswick-Perth Amboy-Sayreville area of New Jersey. The five next most affluent areas will be Grand Forks, N.D.; Nassau-Suffolk Counties, N.Y.; the Pascagoula-Moss Point area of Mississippi; metropolitan Newark, N.J.; and Ann Arbor, Mich.

Which should you choose—the higher need for doctors or the local population's ability to pay? I say you've got to give equal weight to each factor. And that's just what I've done in putting together a system or worksheet that provides a "doctor opportunity

FIGURE 4-2 ══════════════════════════════════════════

## Do Your Own Doctor Opportunity Rating (D.O.R.)

| Area: | Example figures | Your figures |
|---|---|---|
| **A.** Office-based private-practice M.D.s: U.S. | 217,730 | ———— |
| **B.** Population: U.S. | 215,881,400 | ———— |
| **C.** Population per doctor: B divided by A | 992 | ———— |
| **D.** Effective buying income | $1,176,240,000,000 | ———— |
| **E.** Per capita income: D divided by B | $5,449 | ———— |
| **F.** Physicians in area of study | 8,198 | ———— |
| **G.** Population in area | 7,344,800 | ———— |
| **H.** Population per doctor: G divided by F | 896 | ———— |
| **I.** Effective buying income | $46,478,000,000 | ———— |
| **J.** Per capita income: I divided by G | $6,328 | ———— |
| **K.** Relative need for doctors (percentage of U.S.): H divided by C times 100 | 90 | ———— |
| **L.** Relative ability to pay doctors (percentage of U.S.): J divided by E times 100 | 116 | ———— |
| **M.** D.O.R. (U.S.: 100): K + L divided by 2 | 103 | ———— |

rating" (D.O.R.) for any state, county, or city for which one can find the necessary raw data—population, personal income, and the number of physicians in office-based private practice.

Using the U.S. as the measuring post—a rating of 100 on the D.O.R.—you can see where any area stands, given the necessary data. Figure 4-1 gives the D.O.R. for each state and the District of Columbia, and Figure 4-2 shows you how to arrive at the D.O.R. for the area that interests you. But let me skip past all that detail here and get to the significant stuff.

Alaska, for example. It's important because it stands at the top of the ratings among the 50 states and the District of Columbia. It's not just affluent, as we've seen; it also needs more physicians. Its D.O.R. is 149 on a scale that establishes 100 as the norm.

The practical value of the D.O.R. is that it indicates where the best opportunities for private practice are likely to be found. But remember that it's an indication—nothing more. Within any state, good opportunities may be found. In preparing the research for this chapter, I asked my staff to do D.O.R.s for five states, picked at random, except that they're from the corners of the U.S. Later, I discovered that all five are in or near the lower 20 per cent on the state D.O.R. list. Yet all, including low-rated Arizona, have counties

*(Continued on page 50)*

FIGURE 4-3 ═══════════════════════════════════════════

## Doctor Opportunity Ratings for Arizona (by County)

Equal weight is given to the need for doctors and to patients' ability to pay for medical services. U.S.: 100.

| | | | |
|---|---|---|---|
| Apache | 333 | **United States** | **100** |
| Graham | 205 | | |
| Navajo | 177 | Mohave | 98 |
| Pinal | 157 | Coconino | 96 |
| Gila | 156 | Yavapai | 93 |
| Cochise | 142 | State of Arizona | 87 |
| Santa Cruz | 140 | Maricopa | 86 |
| Greenlee | 133 | Pima | 80 |
| Yuma | 111 | | |

FIGURE 4-4

## Doctor Opportunity Ratings
## for Florida (by County)

Equal weight is given to the need for doctors and to patients' ability to pay for medical services. U.S.: 100.

| | | | |
|---|---|---|---|
| Holmes | 358 | Hamilton | 117 |
| Bradford | 317 | St. Lucie | 115 |
| Gilchrist | 294 | De Soto | 113 |
| Sumter | 284 | Columbia | 109 |
| Suwannee | 220 | Marion | 107 |
| Madison | 216 | | |
| Washington | 196 | **United States** | **100** |
| Dixie | 194 | | |
| Levy | 190 | Brevard | 99 |
| Jackson | 184 | St. Johns | 98 |
| Jefferson | 180 | Manatee | 98 |
| Walton | 179 | Hillsborough | 97 |
| Calhoun | 168 | Lake | 96 |
| Baker | 164 | Collier | 95 |
| Santa Rosa | 160 | Duval | 95 |
| Franklin | 159 | Charlotte | 94 |
| Putnam | 155 | Palm Beach | 93 |
| Nassau | 153 | Lee | 93 |
| Union | 152 | Polk | 93 |
| Taylor | 152 | Leon | 93 |
| Okaloosa | 145 | Monroe | 92 |
| Gadsen | 144 | Escambia | 92 |
| Wakulla | 142 | Broward | 92 |
| Hendry | 136 | Pinellas | 91 |
| Seminole | 133 | State of Florida | 91 |
| Citrus | 131 | Orange | 90 |
| Pasco | 131 | Flagler | 88 |
| Gulf | 131 | Sarasota | 86 |
| Osceola | 126 | Volusia | 86 |
| Hernando | 126 | Indian River | 86 |
| Okeechobee | 122 | Dade | 85 |
| Clay | 119 | Highlands | 83 |
| Hardee | 119 | Alachua | 72 |
| Bay | 119 | | |

of unusually high potential. In those five states you'll find 11 counties with D.O.R. ratings above 200.

Florida is especially interesting. It's 48th on the state D.O.R. listing, yet it has 20 counties with ratings above 150, including six that are above 200. Dade and Palm Beach counties aren't among those top-raters, so don't head for Miami or West Palm Beach expecting to find instant wealth and adoration no matter where in town you hang your shingle. Dade and Palm Beach counties, despite their fabled wealth, score under 100. So if you do go there, you'd better have a specific opportunity awaiting.

That's good advice for any under-100 area. But we both know that professional opportunity also depends on such factors as specialty, association, individual skill, and circumstances. My purpose in going to all the bother of putting together D.O.R. tables isn't to guarantee success or failure but simply to indicate the more likely places for a hopeful new practitioner to look for an opportunity.

In this day of Medicaid, Medicare, and an impending national health-insurance plan, does it really make any sense to give ability to pay equal weighting with doctor-patient ratios? My rationale is this: We still don't know what form national health insurance will take, and the Medicaid-Medicare programs have become decreasingly significant factors in many practitioners' incomes. In

FIGURE 4-5 ══════════════════════════════════════════════

## Doctor Opportunity Ratings for Maine (by County)

Equal weight is given to the need for doctors and to patients' ability to pay for medical services. U.S.: 100.

| | | | |
|---|---|---|---|
| Waldo | 147 | Androscoggin | 93 |
| Washington | 135 | State of Maine | 91 |
| Piscataquis | 119 | Hancock | 91 |
| Franklin | 117 | Kennebec | 90 |
| Somerset | 111 | Penobscot | 89 |
| Arroostook | 109 | Lincoln | 88 |
| Sagadahoc | 103 | Cumberland | 81 |
| York | 102 | Knox | 80 |
| **United States** | **100** | | |

some states, Medicaid pays less and less and gets around to paying ever more slowly, year after year. In some communities, it's becoming hard to find a doctor who will accept new Medicaid patients. Never mind, for now, the social implications of that fact; we're talking here only about Medicaid as a financial factor. Medicare is generally a better-run, more financially significant program, but I'm having trouble thinking of more than three practices that would clearly miss that program if it suddenly disappeared.

In other words, I believe a community's ability to pay for medical services is still as important as its need for doctors in determining how much of an opportunity it offers.

But how are you to determine the relative opportunity of a county not covered in the five-state D.O.R. tables found in this chapter? Use the worksheet in Figure 4-2. For raw population and income data, you can subscribe to S&MM (originally Sales &

FIGURE 4-6 ══════════════════════════════════════════

## Doctor Opportunity Ratings for New Mexico (by County)

Equal weight is given to the need for doctors and to patients' ability to pay for medical services. U.S.: 100.

| | | | |
|---|---|---|---|
| Hidalgo | 332 | Rio Arriba | 109 |
| Mora | 276 | Eddy | 107 |
| Valencia | 209 | Dona Ana | 107 |
| Luna | 191 | Taos | 106 |
| Torrance | 187 | Union | 104 |
| McKinley | 171 | | |
| Catron | 163 | **United States** | **100** |
| Sandoval | 149 | | |
| Otero | 139 | Colfax | 99 |
| Quay | 137 | Chaves | 98 |
| Roosevelt | 133 | Los Almamos | 96 |
| Lea | 123 | State of New Mexico | 95 |
| Curry | 122 | Sierra | 94 |
| San Juan | 121 | San Miguel | 90 |
| Lincoln | 119 | De Baca | 81 |
| Grant | 118 | Bernalillo | 80 |
| Guadalupe | 114 | Santa Fe | 72 |
| Socorro | 110 | | |

## Getting started in private practice

Marketing Management) for $22 a year, published at 633 Third Ave., New York 10017. It prints special issues in July and October that provide current estimates and five-year projections for every county and metropolitan area in the nation. (It's the source of those growth predictions made earlier in this chapter.)

Unfortunately, the doctor counts are harder to come by. An excellent source, when freshly updated, is the paperback "Physician Distribution and Medical Licensure in the U.S.," published by the Center for Health Services Research and Development, American Medical Association. The latest edition available as this book is being prepared offers information for 1976. For purposes of this chapter, the A.M.A. kindly allowed me access to fresh, computerized doctor counts (including both M.D.s and D.O.s and both A.M.A. members and nonmembers) maintained for the society by Fisher-Stevens, Inc., Clifton, N.J.

FIGURE 4-7 ═══════════════════════════════════════

### Doctor Opportunity Ratings for Oregon (by County)

Equal weight is given to the need for doctors and to patients' ability to pay for medical services. U.S.: 100.

| | | | |
|---|---|---|---|
| Columbia | 185 | Tillamook | 86 |
| Curry | 172 | Umatilla | 85 |
| Grant | 153 | Wallowa | 84 |
| Polk | 146 | Union | 84 |
| Baker | 111 | Josephine | 84 |
| Lincoln | 109 | Clakamas | 84 |
| Jefferson | 108 | Douglas | 83 |
| Washington | 107 | Lake | 79 |
| Crock | 101 | Morrow | 78 |
| | | Lane | 77 |
| **United States** | **100** | Wasco | 76 |
| | | Marion | 76 |
| Harney | 98 | Coos | 74 |
| Hood River | 94 | Jackson | 70 |
| State of Oregon | 92 | Clatsop | 70 |
| Yamhill | 91 | Deschutes | 69 |
| Klamath | 88 | Multnomah | 62 |
| Malheur | 87 | Benton | 57 |
| Linn | 86 | | |

Don't bother writing to Fisher-Stevens, but do take the time to send a note to the A.M.A.'s Order Department (535 North Dearborn St., Chicago 60610), asking when "Physician Distribution" will again be updated. By the time you're reading these words, perhaps a new edition will be ready.

Your alternative is to ask county or state societies of special interest to you for their own estimates of their office-based physician population. (Unless you're a pathologist or other hospital-based specialist, the opportunity indication you seek is more closely related to the office-based crowd than to an overall count.) You can still use the worksheet in Figure 4-2 and come up with at least an idea of the relative opportunities in the places that interest you. And, of course, you don't necessarily need to subscribe to S&MM; your university or public library may have it on file.

Another book, "Handbook of Medical Specialties," sells for $16.95 in hardcover and $9.95 in paperback and is published by Human Sciences Press, 72 Fifth Ave., New York 10011. It will give you some specialty counts that may suggest how much need there is for your specialty in a given area. Henry Wechsler, Ph.D., the director of research for The Medical Foundation, Inc., in Boston, wrote the book. He tells you, for instance, that Washington, D.C., has more specialists per thousand of population than any of the 50 states and yet may offer excellent opportunities for plastic surgeons, who are in short supply. The book provides evidence, too, that Florida, only 18th on the list in all specialties, has very little need for more plastic surgeons, cardiologists, or urologists and that Idaho, North Dakota, and Alabama, though right at the bottom in supply of specialists in general, enjoy above-average representation in some specialties—pulmonary disease and ophthalmology in Idaho, for instance.

For about $48, then, you can acquire your own three-source study. S&MM updates its data once yearly; the A.M.A.'s "Distribution" is corrected every year or two (the 1977 edition cost $15.95); "Handbook of Medical Specialties," first published in 1976, will be updated as sales warrant, the publisher says.

Once you've narrowed your probable locations down to three or two with the help of those sources and the D.O.R. worksheet—and then to one on the basis of personal visits and inter-views—you'll be ready to seek out your own private office.

Forget about trying to set up an office in your home (an arrangement whose time has passed). Instead, look for space in an office as close as possible to your hospital in the best medical building on doctors' row—or, at least, the best one you can afford. Then follow the suggestions you'll find in Chapter 8.

But first take the trouble to go through all this work to find the right place. Practice where you're needed. That's as basic a rule of good practice management as there is. If you come away from this book with only one idea, let it be that one.

# 5

## Start right in with a friend or two? Could work!

In the last chapter, we discussed how to find a location where your services are needed. In doing so, you may very well run into one or more attractive locations that could support two or three new doctors or even more. If you've gone through training with a compatible friend or two, there's no reason in the world why you shouldn't consider going into practice together in exactly that kind of location.

The chances are that your friends—for the balance of this chapter, let's keep things simple and assume there will be three of you—are in the same specialty. That's just as well. Small, single-specialty groups seem to work more smoothly than small, mixed-specialty groups. Coverage is one reason; an internist may not be too thrilled about covering for a pediatrician. Referral problems are another reason; the competing family practitioners in town won't be too thrilled with the idea of referring patients to a surgeon with a family practitioner-partner.

# Getting started in private practice

Partner? I'll use the term "partner" throughout the rest of this chapter—but not because I'll be thinking of the word in the legal or tax sense. Maybe you'll be incorporated. Maybe one of you will be the proprietor, and the others will be the employees. The differences between a partnership and a professional corporation or a proprietorship are basically two: real and imagined. The second of those differences is significant only if you let it be. The real difference lies simply with the income tax forms you file—Form 1065 for a partnership, Form 1120 for a corporation, Schedule C with Form 1040 for a proprietorship. Big deal? No.

An optional difference is attitude. People have all sorts of funny notions about the three ways of doing business, and those ideas serve very little purpose. In fact, they can get in the way of some very effective, tax-attractive arrangements. What's the solution? Change your attitude.

Take partnership. A lot of people mistakenly think the term means that income after expenses is shared in equal parts. Not so. Of three partners, one may be entitled to 90 per cent of the net, a second to 9 per cent, and a third to 1 per cent. But for what? Labor? Capital contributed? The three partners need not put in equal amounts of capital.

The same goes for a professional corporation. The three of you need not be equal shareholders. Each of you can be compensated fairly without regard to the number of shares you own. As the boss, you can set policy and hire and fire and, if you have enough shares of stock, keep your two shareholder-colleagues from ganging up on you and throwing you out. But that's the advantage of being an *owner*. It has very little to do with the reason doctors incorporate. Mostly, they do so in order to become employees of the corporation, since the tax benefits arise from being an employee, not from being a shareholder.

If you understand that, you understand more about a professional corporation (P.C.) than many of your older colleagues do. Many of them just don't seem to realize that a P.C. is a completely separate tax entity, like another person—not just more initials to add after one's name, like some kind of supplemental college degree. I've seen doctors sign personal correspondence with their

names and the initials M.D. and then add the initials P.C. Corporations may be tax entities, but they can't write, and they can't sign
their names.

As an employee of a professional corporation, whether you
happen to be a shareholder or not, you qualify just like any other
employee for the employee fringe-benefit plans—the retirement
plan, for example. That's the baby, remember, that's going to make
America rich.

You can just as easily qualify for a retirement plan in a
proprietorship or a partnership. As either a proprietor-employee or
a partner-employee, you qualify to participate in a Keogh retirement plan and can, under usual circumstances, invest or save as
much as $7,500 a year tax-free. But as an employee in a profes-
sional corporation, you can participate fully in all your employee-
benefit plans; you can, for instance, invest as much as $28,175 a
year in a retirement plan tax-free.

No matter which of the three ways to practice you elect, you
and your two partners will share expenses. When many of your
older colleagues hear the words "expense sharing" they immediately have visions of solo practitioners sharing such common space
as the reception room and the business office, with each paying for
his own space for examining rooms, consultation rooms, and the
like. But expense sharing is automatic, whether the three of you
practice that way or as partners or in a P.C. I mean, if the three of
you share the income, who do you think is sharing the expenses?

Understanding what you're doing may be the least of your
problems. Many of your elders' practices have broken up because
of jealousy, frequently because one partner took extra time off.

If the extra helping is unfair, then it's no wonder someone got
upset. You can be paid in two ways, in time or in money. If by prior
agreement you and I, partners, are paid the same amount of
money from our partnership and if your productivity brings in 10
times more money than mine does, then you *ought* to be upset with
me, and you probably ought to bust up the partnership if I take
more time-off than you do. On the other hand, I shouldn't be upset
if you take more time off than I do—not, at least, until your extra
time off drags your fee production down to a level below mine.

But that sort of arrangement—forcing the big producer to take time off—never happens. Practices break up first, all because someone got the idea that partnership means equal pay regardless of fee production. But why equal pay? Isn't it more logical to pay each in proportion to what he brings in?

Now, there are two basic ways to compensate partners. I call one way tenure, the other production. Those share-and-share-alike arrangements follow the tenure route; to get an equal cut of the income pie, you need to attain tenure by putting in three years or whatever with the group. A production arrangement links compensation to productivity. There are variations on those themes, actually mixtures of them that are commonly called point systems, but the real ingredients are those two. The most common production-based arrangement is for partners to share the net income (after the office expenses are paid) in proportion to each doctor's production. That way, both the overhead and the net income are shared in proportion to production.

A more sophisticated version is to share the overhead in proportion to production and to share the net income in proportion to gross income brought in by each doctor. After all, production is production whether it's paid for or not and thus is a measure of office expense, rather than income. Then, too, one partner's collection ratio may vary enormously from another's. You, bless you, always refer a patient with a routine question about fees to our financial secretary. But I, seeking community acclaim as the nicer guy, make a point of replying to any such inquiry with a suggestion that the patient not worry about the fee, and, of course, he won't. So, if we bother to keep score, we may discover that the payments for services rendered by you in any given 12-month period total an amount equal to 90 per cent of your production for the same period. (That's what a collection ratio is: gross practice income expressed as a percentage of production in a 12-month period.) But, since I have that knack of so grandly giving our money away, my collection ratio may come to no more than 60 per cent. In our practice, then, the need for that more sophisticated compensation arrangement seems obvious.

Besides, who's to say that I shouldn't give away my services?

If I were in solo practice, I could give away what I wished. Why should things be any different just because you're my partner? Indeed, I should have that right. So should you. So should any partner. Anyone in a multidoctor practice should have the same rights and privileges he'd have in solo practice. Any doctor who has fewer rights and privileges is needlessly restricted. All he needs is a compensation arrangement under which payments are credited to the doctor who did the work, while office overhead is apportioned in proportion to each doctor's production. That's fair.

Compensation? Well, there are two kinds—direct and indirect. At least, there are two kinds for doctors who qualify for employee benefits, as in a professional corporation. Let's assume, to illustrate how this works, that you and your two partners each expect to produce $60,000 worth of services in your first year. Let's be reasonably conservative and figure that your collection ratio in that year will run 85 per cent, which means that your gross practice income for each man will total only $51,000. Let's assume that basic overhead will take half that amount, leaving a compensation fund of $25,500 for each physician.

Don't plan to give up the full $25,500 as salary. Better plan on paying a salary of about 75 per cent of the projected compensation. That works out to $19,125, nominally $796.875 a payday, assuming two paydays a month, 24 paydays a year. But let's hedge the bets even further. Let's cut each man's salary back to $625 a payday, which works out to an annual rate of $15,000, and keep it there for, say, six months. At that point, you can look at the numbers for each physician and reassess your financial situation.

Even in six months, you may see clear trends developing— Dr. A right on his $60,000 production target and his $51,000 gross practice income target, Dr. B doing better, Dr. C doing not nearly as well. Thus, Dr. A can still look forward to receiving a total of $19,125 for the year. He's already received $7,500 at the time of the six-month reassessment, leaving $11,625 in salary to be paid during the remaining six months of the first year—$968.75 for each remaining payday. Fine. He gets a salary increase. So does Dr. B. Dr. C. doesn't. He may even need to take a cut or to give up all thoughts of a bonus or other fringe benefits.

FIGURE 5-1 ═══════════════════════════════════════

## How Much Working Capital to Launch a Practice and How to Reward It

How much working capital is required varies widely from one situation to another, depending largely on the practice's immediate income potential; the figures below are representative. The number of shares to be issued by a professional corporation is not often significant; at Line B, 100 shares for each doctor may be assumed, though the distribution might just as easily be 300 shares for one doctor and 100 for the other or some other distribution, such as 200 shares for each. The dividend indicated at Line C can be as the owners agree. The multiplier at Line D depends on the applicable corporate tax rate in effect at the time; it's subject to change. The total shown at Line F should match that at Line C.

|  | Example figures | Your figures | Line |
|---|---|---|---|
| **A.** Working capital required: | | | |
| Rent: 3 months or _____ months: | $ 4,900 | _____ | |
| Equipment lease: 6 months or _____ months: | $ 5,145 | _____ | |
| Staff wages: 3 months or _____ months: | $ 5,200 | _____ | |
| Loan repayment: Malpractice insurance: 3 months or _____ months: | $ 2,200 | _____ | |
| Loan repayment: Doctors' salaries: 3 months or _____ months: | $ 12,000 | _____ | |
| Slush fund: | $ 3,000 | _____ | |
| TOTAL: | $ 32,445 | _____ | A |
| **B.** Shares issued | 200 | _____ | B |
| **C.** Annual dividend to be paid: Line A multiplied by: □.10 □.15 □.20 □.25 □._____ | $3,244.50 | _____ | C |
| **D.** Taxable net corporation income required: Line C multiplied by 1.25 or _____ | $4,055.63 | _____ | D |
| **E.** Annual dividend per share: Line C divided by Line B | $ 16.2225 | _____ | E |

**F.** Each doctor's shareholdings and total dividend payment (shares multiplied by Line E):

| Doctor | Shares owned | Dividend payment |
|---|---|---|
| _____ | _____ | _____ |
| _____ | _____ | _____ |
| _____ | _____ | _____ |
| _____ | _____ | _____ |
| TOTAL:· $3,244.50 | _____ | F |

Remember, Dr. A is still projecting total compensation of $25,500, and reasonably so. But his salary will provide only 75 per cent, $19,125. Thus, he can take the difference of $6,375 as a bonus. Or he can take both a bonus and a benefit—say, reimbursement of the health-insurance premiums he paid during the year and of the money he paid the orthodontist. The health-expense-reimbursement benefit may come to, say, $1,375, leaving him with $5,000 for a cash end-of-year bonus. And, instead of reporting the full $25,500 on his Form W-2 and paying taxes on that amount, he'll have to report only $24,125. Money paid out in a corporation's employee health-expense-reimbursement plan is tax-deductible by the corporation as a business expense.

Now that they've got labor's reward settled, just what are they to pay for the use of capital? Well, how much capital is there in this corporation? And how much capital equipment is on the books? All sorts of rules of thumb are being used to determine how much reward needs to go or should go to capital each year, but one rule is an amount equal to 10 per cent of the money invested in the professional corporations. The payment will be in the form of a dividend, which must come from the corporation's after-tax net income. To figure out what the pretax net income is, multiply the dividend by 1.25—for example, a $3,000 dividend multiplied by 1.25 equals $3,750. The Federal tax is 20 per cent, so multiply $3,750 by 0.20, which equals $750 in tax and leaves $3,000 for the dividend. Figure 5-1 includes all the working arithmetic, including a start-up budget guide.

How many shares of stock are outstanding? Whatever the number, divide it into the $3,000 to determine the dividend share.

Since there are three physicians in the practice, must they contribute capital in equal amounts, $10,000 each? Not at all. If Dr. A is rich and Drs. B and C have all their money tied up in debts, then Dr. A can put up the whole $30,000. Of course, he'll get all the outstanding shares of stock—say, 300 shares, worth $100 each. That way, all the dividends will go to him. Fair enough.

But Drs. B and C may not be too tickled with the idea of having all the stock in Dr. A's safe-deposit box, since policy in a corporation is determined by vote—one vote a share. So Drs. B and C may offer, in a written agreement accepted by Dr. A before he even puts up the money, to purchase at some reasonable future time (by a given deadline) up to one-third of Dr. A's holdings. Or each may agree that he *must* purchase his third by a given date. Or each may buy his shares then and there, giving Dr. A a promissory note for the money due.

A written agreement is necessary for three reasons: First, it provides a written record of the terms of the agreement, which sure beats memory; second, it gives all parties some evidence that may be needed to arbitrate their differences later; and, third, it spells out the terms of a professional divorce if the practice breaks up. This last point is the most important one. Going in, you need to have agreements on who gets to stay in the office (high card); who's to get custody of the patients' records (each doctor gets the charts of those patients he normally sees); whether or not the telephone number is to remain in force (change it); and what's to be done about the accounts receivable (in a productivity-based arrangement, just pay out the money due each doctor as his patients pay for the services he's rendered, subtracting 20 per cent for billing and collection expenses).

How to keep track of everything? It's really quite easy. Whenever a service is rendered to a patient, whether in the office or out, a charge slip or some other record goes from the doctor to the financial secretary. The day's fees can be totaled on the daysheet, one column for each doctor. And when each patient's fee is posted to his ledger card, the doctor who provided the services can be identified by initial.

Whenever a payment for services is received, the amount paid is entered on the patient's ledger card. At that time it's an easy matter for the financial secretary to look at the card and determine which doctor provided the service that's being paid for. Then she enters the payment on the daysheet. There's a separate column there for each doctor's payments. These columns, too, are totaled at the end of the day.

How should you handle a partial payment by a patient who's been seen by two or more doctors? It goes in payment of the oldest debt owing.

If you're receiving computer-billing services, the computer may be programmed to keep the score for you—both fees and payments. All the computer-billing service firms do allocate the production, but not all sort out the payments. The better ones do.

My recommendation? Do enter practice with a friend or two if you can find a place that truly needs your services. Just avoid the problems that have torn other groups apart. As we've just seen, that's not impossible.

# 6

# Start-up red tape and paperwork: Not so difficult

A licensed physician in my state, New Jersey, is required to have completed four years of medical school and one year of an approved internship. The licensing fee is $150, whether the license is obtained through a Federation of State Medical Boards examination and endorsement (also known as FLEX, for Federation Licensing Exam), endorsement of the National Board of Medical Examiners, or endorsement of a sister state license.

The rules are probably different in the state in which you plan to practice, since the requirements and the fees vary from state to state. In Kentucky, for instance, the fee for the state medical board examination is $125, and the licensing fee is $125. In Minnesota, an examination application costs $125, a reciprocal application costs $100, and there's an annual registration fee of $20. In California, a license must be renewed every other year at a cost of $20. In New Jersey, the biennial registration fee is $30.

I mention New Jersey again not just because I happen to live there, but because that state is probably the nation's leader in new efforts to police doctors—an effort that undoubtedly traces its cause to the increase in the 1970s in public concern about medical malpractice. Until 1972, the New Jersey Board of Medical Examiners was, like many other such boards, headed by a physician who

FIGURE 6-1 ═══════════════════════════════════════════

## Basic Information Supplied by the
## Michigan Medical Practice Board

Authority for medical licensure and regulation is vested in the Michigan Medical Practice Board. A copy of the Medical Practice Act, as amended, is enclosed for your information. The fee for initial licensure is $105.00 and the annual reregistration fee is $25.00.

The following is basic information about the procedures to be followed by candidates for Michigan licensure to practice medicine.

### A. Graduates of American Medical Schools

1. The Michigan Medical Practice Act requires that an applicant for a license must be a graduate of a medical college and must have completed one year of postgraduate medical education at an approved hospital. That one year may be part of a longer residency training program.
2. The Michigan Medical Practice Board issues a "temporary license" to the medical school graduate during his first year of postgraduate education. This license may be renewed annually for a term not to exceed five years.
3. The new doctor who wants to practice in Michigan must pass either the "National Boards" examination or the "FLEX" examination. The "National Boards" is administered by the National Board of Medical Examiners at medical school locations. The FLEX examination is a project of the Federation of State Licensing Boards of the United States. The letters FLEX stand for Federation Licensing Examination.
4. The Michigan Medical Practice Board offers the FLEX examination twice each year. The examination is divided into three parts. An applicant for a Michigan license may take one or two parts of the test over a second time, but if he fails one part a second time, he then must take the entire test over.
5. Physicians who hold licenses in other states may apply for a Michigan license through reciprocity. Certain provisions must be met.

### B. Graduates of Foreign Medical Schools

1. Graduates of foreign medical schools must take the ECFMG examination before they can begin to qualify for a Michigan license to practice medicine. The ECFMG examination is a project of the Educational Council for Foreign Medical Graduates, which is sponsored by the AMA, American Hospital

served as a part-time secretary. But then, along about the time a new state deputy attorney general took a special interest in investigating health-care complaints, the state found funds for a full-time executive secretary. In 1975, of the 125 medical licenses lifted across the country, 23 belonged to New Jersey doctors.

*(Continued on page 70)*

Association, Association of American Colleges, Association for Hospital and Medical Education, and the Federation of State Medical Boards of the United States. (Graduates of Canadian or Puerto Rican medical schools are not required to obtain certification from ECFMG because Canadian medical schools are accredited by the Liaison Committee on Medical Education, just as are the medical schools in the U.S. and Puerto Rico.)

2. The ECFMG examination is given twice each year at various locations across the nation and around the world. The Michigan center is Ann Arbor.
3. The examination is divided into two parts, a medical part and an English part. The candidate may take either part over if he or she fails to get a passing grade.
4. Once the foreign medical graduate has passed the ECFMG, then he must go through the same Michigan licensing procedures that graduates of American medical schools must complete—one year of postgraduate training at an approved hospital and then a passing grade on the National Boards or the FLEX examination.

For further information or application **for** Michigan licensure contact:

Mr. Bert C. Brennan, Exec. Dir.
Michigan Medical Practice Board
1033 South Washington Avenue
Lansing, MI 48926
(517) 373-0680

Of assistance to physicians wishing to practice in Michigan is the Physicians' Placement Service, operated by the Michigan Health Council with the cooperation of the Michigan State Medical Society. The Service is offered to physicians and to communities free of charge through special financial grants from The Upjohn Company of Kalamazoo, the Michigan State Medical Society, Blue Cross and Blue Shield of Michigan, several Michigan foundations, and many community hospitals, clinics, and individuals.

For information contact:

Physicians' Placement Service
Michigan Health Council
P.O. Box 1010
East Lansing, MI 48823
(517) 337-1615

FIGURE 6-2 =====================================================

## Where to Write for a State-License Application

☐ Alabama Board of Medical Examiners, Box 946, Montgomery 36102.
☐ Alaska Department of Commerce, Division of Occupational Licensing, Pouch D, Juneau 99801.
☐ Arizona Board of Medical Examiners, 810 West Bethany Home Rd., Phoenix 85013.
☐ Arkansas Board of Medical Examiners, Box 102, Harrisburg 72432.
☐ California Board of Medical Examiners, 1020 N St., Room A-202, Sacramento 95814.
☐ Canal Zone Director of Health, Box M, Balboa Heights 00101.
☐ Colorado Board of Medical Examiners, 1612 Tremont Pl., Denver 80202.
☐ Connecticut Board of Medical Examiners, 79 Elm St., Hartford 06115
☐ Delaware Board of Medical Examiners, Jesse S. Cooper Bldg., Dover 19901.
☐ District of Columbia Commission on Licensure, 614 H St., N.W., Washington, D.C. 20001.
☐ Florida Board of Medical Examiners, 305 Blount St., Tallahassee 32301.
☐ Georgia Board of Medical Examiners, 166 Pryor St. S.W., Atlanta 30303.
☐ Guam Board of Medical Examiners, Box AX, Agana 96910.
☐ Hawaii Department of Regulatory Agencies, Box 8469, Honolulu 96801.
☐ Idaho Board of Medical Examiners, 407 West Bannosh St., Boise 83702.
☐ Illinois Superintendent of Registration, 628 East Adams St., Springfield 62704.
☐ Indiana Board of Health, 1375 West 16th St., Indianapolis 46202.
☐ Iowa Board of Medical Examiners, 910 Insurance Exchange Bldg., Des Moines 50309.
☐ Kansas Board of Medical Examiners, 292 New Brotherhood Bldg., Kansas City 66010.
☐ Kentucky Board of Medical Examiners, 3532 Ephraim McDowell Dr., Louisville 40205.
☐ Louisiana Board of Medical Examiners, 621 Hibernia Bank Bldg., New Orleans 70112.
☐ Maine Board of Medical Examiners, 100 College Ave., Waterville 04901.
☐ Maryland Board of Medical Examiners, 201 West Preston St., Baltimore 21201.
☐ Massachusetts Board of Medical Examiners, 100 Cambridge St., Boston 02202.
☐ Michigan Medical Practice Board, 1033 South Washington Ave., Lansing 48926.
☐ Minnesota Board of Medical Examiners, 200 South Robert St., Suite 203, St. Paul 55107.
☐ Mississippi Board of Medical Examiners, Box 1700, Jackson 39205.

☐ Missouri Board of Medical Examiners, Box 4, Jefferson City 65101.

☐ Montana Board of Medical Examiners, Lalonde Bldg. No. 4, Helena 59601.

☐ Nebraska Bureau of Examining Boards, Department of Health, 1003 O St., Lincoln 68509.

☐ Nevada Board of Medical Examiners, 1281 Terminal Way No. 211, Reno 89502.

☐ New Hampshire Board of Medical Examiners, 61 South Spring St., Concord 03301.

☐ New Jersey Board of Medical Examiners, 28 West State St., Trenton 08625.

☐ New Mexico Board of Medical Examiners, 210 East March St., Santa Fe 87501.

☐ New York Board of Medical Examiners, 99 Washington Ave., Albany 12210.

☐ North Carolina Board of Medical Examiners, 222 North Person St., Suite 214, Raleigh 27601.

☐ North Dakota Board of Medical Examiners, Box 1198, Bismarck 58501.

☐ Ohio Board of Medical Examiners, 21 Broad St., Columbus 43215.

☐ Oklahoma Board of Medical Examiners, 3013 Northwest 59th St., Oklahoma City 73112.

☐ Oregon Board of Medical Examiners, 317 Southwest Alder St., Portland 97204.

☐ Pennsylvania Board of Medical Examiners, 279 Boas St., Harrisburg 17120.

☐ Puerto Rico Board of Medical Examiners, Box 3271, San Juan 00907.

☐ Rhode Island Board of Medical Examiners, Health Dept. Bldg., Davis St., Providence 02908.

☐ South Carolina Board of Medical Examiners, 1315 Blanding St., Columbia 29201.

☐ South Dakota Board of Medical Examiners, 608 West Avenue North, Sioux Falls 57104.

☐ Tennessee Board of Medical Examiners, 350 Capitol Hill Bldg., Nashville 37219.

☐ Texas Board of Medical Examiners, 900 Southwest Tower, Austin 78701.

☐ Utah Board of Medical Examiners, 330 East Fourth St., Salt Lake City 84111.

☐ Vermont Board of Medical Examiners, 126 State St., Montpelier 05602.

☐ Virginia Board of Medical Examiners, 505 Washington St., Suite 200, Portsmouth 23704.

☐ Virgin Islands Board of Medical Examiners, Box 1442, St. Thomas 00801.

☐ Washington Board of Medical Examiners, Box 649, Olympia 98504.

☐ West Virginia Board of Medical Examiners, 1800 Washington St., Charleston 25305.

☐ Wisconsin Board of Medical Examiners, 201 East Washington Ave., Madison 53702.

☐ Wyoming Board of Medical Examiners, State Office Bldg., Cheyenne 82001.

## Getting started in private practice

Now, at least in New Jersey, a complaint by a patient or a hospital administrator or a colleague won't lie unnoticed on some overworked board member's desk. It will very likely get as much attention as it deserves. Any doctor who indiscriminately dispenses narcotics faces a strong probability of having his license lifted, at the least. Illegal drug use also stands to be punished by the board, as does aberrant or deviant behavior indicating psychiatric problems or incompetence brought about by advanced age. The board not only suspends and revokes licenses but also levies fines for a variety of reasons, ranging from fraudulent advertising to practicing in a hospital without a proper license.

To apply for a license to practice, you need to write to the state board of medical examiners. You get back an application and instructions—and perhaps more. In Michigan, the Medical Practice Board, as the examiners are called there, sends along a copy of the state's Medical Practice Act plus a two-page summary of the basic information you need to know. Those two pages are reproduced in this chapter (see Figure 6-1). Similarly, the Minnesota State Board of Medical Examiners sends along a copy of its rules and regulations. Whatever your state sends you, take the time to read it; you may find a totally unexpected requirement. For instance, in Minne-

FIGURE 6-3 ═══════════════════════════════════════════

### Checklisting the Ethical and Legal Requirements

☐ Write to the state's board of medical examiners for an application for a license to practice medicine. Also, ask if a state narcotics license is required. Request a copy of the state's medical practices act.

☐ Write for an application for a Federal narcotics license to the Drug Enforcement Administration, U.S. Department of Justice, Box 28083, Central Station, Washington, D.C. 20005.

☐ Phone your community's tax collector and ask if you need a business license.

☐ Call the local office of the Internal Revenue Service and ask for Form SS-4, the application for an employer identification number.

☐ Send your county medical society an advance copy of the proposed newspaper announcement of your office's opening.

sota, any professional corporation launched in the state must be registered and must file an annual report with the board.

All state boards are responsible for setting professional standards and policy, preparing and conducting examinations, considering applications, initiating investigations of alleged violations of the state medical practice act and other laws under its jurisdiction, issuing citations, and holding hearings on disciplinary matters. In general, a board may revoke a license to practice, reprimand a physician publicly or in private, or take any other disciplinary actions it considers appropriate.

It's no surprise that a board can take action against demonstrated negligence and incompetence or a felony committed by a physician. But a board can also take disciplinary action for excessive use of diagnostic facilities, the employment of a physician's assistant without the board's advance approval, the employment of a suspended or unlicensed physician, the willful betrayal of a professional secret, the employment of anyone to procure patients, or the signing of any certificate related to the practice of medicine that you know falsely represents the facts. A good deal of what you may consider matters of morals or ethics is, in fact, also a matter of law. So don't for one minute take your state's board of medical examiners or its medical practice act lightly.

A license to practice is only the first of the licenses you need to look into. You also need a Federal narcotics license and quite possibly, depending on where you practice, a state narcotics license, too. For the Federal license, apply to the Drug Enforcement Administration, U.S. Department of Justice, Box 28083, Central Station, Washington, D.C. 20005. Your state board of medical examiners and state medical society can tell you whether you need to apply for a state narcotics license and, if you do, where to write.

Your narcotics registration number must appear on your prescription form, along with your name, whenever you prescribe a controlled drug such as morphine or codeine. A common mistake is to have the number printed on the prescription forms, making both the forms and your office likely prey for those addicts or pushers who make a business of forging prescriptions. If you don't want to increase your risk of theft, get in the habit of writing both your name

**71**

and your narcotics number on each prescription as you hand it out.

In many communities you also need a business license, but you shouldn't rely even on the executive director of the county medical society for the last word here. Ordinances come and go, and in my county there are 70 elected councils writing and rewriting local laws every week—far too much activity for a county society to follow closely: Usually, the business license fee is only a couple of dollars, but you may risk a hefty fine by not filing the appropriate form. Before you move into your new office, call the local tax collector's office and ask if you'll need a business license.

Also, check your local telephone directory or that of a nearby large city for the local Internal Revenue Service office. You need to

FIGURE 6-4 ════════════════════════════════════════

## How to Announce Your Arrival

A local printer or a medical cataloguer like The Colwell Company (201 Kenyon Rd., Champaign, Ill. 61820) can print a paneled, raised-letter announcement like this one. Your county medical society may be willing to run your envelopes through its addressing machine. At this writing, Colwell charges $35.10 for printing 1,000 announcements measuring 5⅝ by 3⅝ inches, and that price includes unprinted envelopes. Addressing the envelopes may cost another $5—the fee at Bergen County Medical Society, Hackensack, N.J. The same announcement can be reproduced by the local newspaper as a professional advertisement.

---

### John Q. Doktor, M.D.

ANNOUNCES THE OPENING OF HIS OFFICE FOR THE

PRACTICE OF FAMILY MEDICINE

123 MAIN STREET

ANYTOWN, U.S.A. 07666

| OFFICE HOURS | TELEPHONE |
| BY APPOINTMENT | (201) 555-1213 |

---

phone there or drop in for a Form SS-4, an application for an employer identification number. When the I.R.S. processes your application, it will assign you the number and send you a packet of forms and income tax withholding tables which you must use every time you prepare a paycheck.

There's really no point in my going into a description of the various forms and how to fill them out. Everything you'll see is easily handled. Just take the time to read the directions that come with the forms. They're not so complicated. You don't have to hire a tax expert to fill them in for you. Any high school graduate should be able to handle them just fine. The most important thing for you to remember is that the penalties can be enormous, including time in jail, if you fail to follow the directions, especially those with regard to paying payroll taxes on time. It's up to you to withhold and to deposit at a nearby Federally chartered bank each employee's income taxes and Social Security contributions, and you must match (and more) each dollar of Social Security tax withheld from an employee. The amount of money involved is shown in the tables that the I.R.S. gives you.

Plan now to spend an hour with that packet of information when it arrives. It's important for you to invest that much time in understanding it.

It's positively mandatory that you look after all those licenses and tax forms before opening your door to patients. But, of course, there's a good deal more to opening a private practice, as any medical management consultant can tell you. I'm indebted, in fact, to the Society of Medical-Dental Management Consultants and its executive secretary, Dean Van Horn, for the information that provides this checklist:

● *Telephone number.* It can sometimes take several weeks to get your phone installed, so you've got to think ahead about that, too.

"It's generally best to order one number and reserve at least a second," Van Horn, himself a management consultant, advises. "Your phone company will probably let you reserve a number that's in consecutive sequence with the first and hold it in reserve without cost until it's needed. When you have it installed, it should be on a hunting or rotary circuit, so that the second number rings if

**73**

someone dials the first when it's busy. In time, you may find it necessary to have a third and perhaps a fourth line, plus one unlisted private line separated from the others so that it's kept open for your outgoing calls."

When first ordering your phone equipment, ask for the kind with five phone buttons and one red hold button. That way, you'll be all set for quick, easy expansion later. And be sure to have the phone company install an intercom and buzzer on all your office telephones.

● *Office equipment.* If you've already made arrangements for financing your clinical and business-office equipment, your next step is to go shopping for it. (You can use Chapters 18 and 19 as your guide.) Just remember: To get the equipment you really want, rather than the equipment you must settle for, you have to plan far enough ahead to allow it to be ordered and shipped. That can take weeks or even months.

● *Office printing.* The best of what you need is discussed in Chapter 9. You need to allow adequate time for it, too, to be delivered. Delivery of printed material can take just as long as the delivery of photocopiers, typewriters, and other office equipment.

● *Newspaper announcement.* Using Figure 6-4 as your guide, work out your copy for a block display ad. But, before taking it to the newspaper, get it cleared by your county medical society. That, too, may take time, if the executive secretary doesn't have the authority to approve your ad on the spot. It may have to be considered at the next meeting of the society's ethics committee.

● *Bank accounts.* You need more than one bank account: a checking account for personal use and another for business.

It's also a good idea to consider opening an account either at a savings institution or in a no-load money-market fund or a municipal-bond mutual fund. All those accounts pay interest, and all savings accounts and many of the funds allow both deposits and withdrawals without the payment of a fee.

Management man Melvin L. Schultz tells me he's seen doctor-clients build up significant amounts of windfall funds just by keeping checking accounts at a minimum level and as much money as possible in savings accounts. As an incentive, he often advises clients to use the extra interest earned for pure pleasure—an office Christmas party, for instance.

But there's more than banking to be considered in connection with cash:

● *Money handling.* You need two stores of cash in the office. The first is a $50 change fund—one roll of dimes ($5), one roll of quarters ($10), 20 singles, and three fives. That's strictly for making change, so from time to time you'll need to exchange some big bills at the bank for new rolls of coins or smaller bills. But the $50 total should always remain fairly constant.

The second cash supply is a petty-cash fund which we'll discuss in greater detail in Chapter 7. To begin, stock the petty-cash fund the same way as the change fund, and then replenish it from time to time, since it's dipped into whenever something needs to be paid for in cash. That need can vary widely. For instance, in some communities the local postmaster accepts only currency at the postage window—no checks. And some of your deliveries will arrive c.o.d.

Then there's bill-paying—a chore you will probably come to hate, not so much because you're spending your hard-earned money but because it's time-consuming. Many of your elder colleagues have developed the bad habit of writing all checks themselves. That's not necessary; an assistant can be assigned to write the checks, look after the invoices and statements, and prepare everything for your signature. That way, someone else does the worst of the task, and you need only pay attention to what you're signing—watching for mistakes in the amount of the bill and the amount of the check.

Make it your policy to pay bills twice monthly (the 10th and the 25th), suggests Van Horn. But also consider:

● *Office policies.* The system you set up for paying bills and otherwise handling money is just one of the subjects you need to discuss with your medical assistants at the first of your monthly staff meetings—important events that we'll discuss in Chapter 15. Who's to do what and how must also be discussed then.

In preparation for that first meeting, you need to look closely at your state's medical practice act. It tells you what your assistants are legally allowed to do. All sorts of tasks that many doctors consider highly delegable may be covered by your state's laws—administering eyedrops, removing sutures and casts, using an electrocardiograph, taking diagnostic X-rays.

Generalizing about the restrictions on such tasks can be misleading. You may not really need to know the usual situation in regard to intravenous procedures, but you'd better find out what the law in your state is. Some states allow almost anyone to do almost anything under a doctor's direction, but most states are a good deal more restrictive than that. In California, for instance, a nurse must be licensed to administer medication by hypodermic needle or to draw blood, but any doctor's employee may telephone prescriptions to pharmacies if the doctor follows up the phone order within a reasonable time with written evidence of the authorization. One exception: For narcotics there must be a written order in hand.

In California, as elsewhere, syringes must be disposed of so that they cannot be reused. One way is to cut the needles with wire cutters and to dispose of both parts in a big glass jar. When the jar is half filled, throw in a scoop or two of cement (you can buy it in reasonable amounts in hardware stores), and then fill the jar to the top with cold water. Put the lid on, shake, and let sit overnight. The next day, the whole thing can be discarded.

It's important for you to delegate all the tasks that can be delegated legally and to good purpose. Until now, a physician could, at least in many states, do pretty much as he liked. But all that's changing. Boards of medical examiners are starting to pay attention to such matters, and they're starting to get tough.

• *Coverage.* Right from the start, be on the lookout for other solo practitioners who seem to be compatible and who fit the requirements of your coverage arrangement. You may not need to look very hard; chances are that they're looking for you.

• *Business insurance.* You need malpractice coverage, of course, and both office and auto liability insurance—and more. But all that's closely related to your family's financial security, so I think that we ought to discuss it in that context in Chapter 21. Right now, let's get back into the subject of handling money and doing it in such a way that the I.R.S. stays off your back.

# The tax game:
# Not so tough if you're
# reasonably well organized

Here's unexpectedly good news for you: Thanks entirely to Federal tax laws, you're going to be a millionaire. The only catch is that you simply must not blow the opportunity.

You won't have to charge high fees, and you won't have to chisel on your income taxes. Even if your practice is below the average on the income scale, you'll be able to put away enough money in a fully tax-sheltered savings program to build up a fund of more than a million dollars by the time you're 65. In fact, if you're a little bit under the average, you'll have more than a million bucks in your account by age 55 if you get started by the time you're 30.

No, you haven't been singled out for some kind of superspe- ·cial treatment by the Federal Government. Everyone with a good retirement plan will be a millionaire someday—everyone, that is, who's young enough now and gets started early enough. Anyone who's self-employed—butcher, baker, candlestick-maker—can get the job done simply by signing up for a Keogh plan free at any

FIGURE 7-1 ═══════════════════════════════════════

## Labels for
## Your Tax Folders

### Business File

Refunds

Depreciation: purchases of capital
equipment, fixtures, furnishings

Business taxes

Rent

Repairs

Salaries, wages to assistants

Business insurance

Legal, professional fees

Retirement plan

Employee-benefit plans

Interest

Communications: phone, postal

Utilities: light, heat, water

Office cleaning, maintenance
services, supplies

Supplies: clinical

Supplies: business

Equipment repair, maintenance

Car expenses

Convention expenses

Other meeting expenses, including
travel, entertainment

Office temporaries, other
contract labor

Loans, salary advances

Business gifts

Salaries, bonuses to doctors

Banking service

Collection fees

Dues, subscriptions

Lab fees

Equipment rental

Tax: F.I.C.A.

Tax: unemployment

Miscellaneous, other

### Family File

Health insurance

Rx medicine, drugs

Physicians, dentists, nursing care

Hospitalization

Rx eyeglasses, appliances

State, local income taxes

Real estate taxes

Personal property tax

Stock transfer, other
miscellaneous taxes

Interest paid: home mortgage

Interest paid: personal loans, other

Charitable contributions

Miscellaneous: alimony, doctors'
union dues, safe-deposit box,
tax adviser's fee, other

Child-care expenses

Political contributions

Casualty losses: fire, theft,
car accident, other

savings bank or savings and loan association. The going yield for long-term accounts is 8.17 per cent as I write these words. Under Keogh, a self-employed person can put away $7,500 a year, watch the earnings compound totally free of current income taxes, and see the total grow to more than $1,292,300 in 35 years.

Anyone practicing in a corporation can do even better if his retirement plan is a good one. And anyone who owns his own corporation is certainly in a position to see that it is.

Every physician in private practice is eligible for either a Keogh plan or a professional-corporation retirement plan. The average doctor in practice today with a reasonably well-managed practice is in a position to have a million dollars in his retirement account in 20 to 25 years.

We'll get into the details later in this book, but the point to be made in this chapter is simply this: There's no point looking for all kinds of tax angles; you just don't need them anymore. The main thing to remember now is to pay your fair share. You needn't pay a cent more, but, if you're going to be a millionaire someday anyway, there's just no point trying to pay a cent less.

The main thing that you need to do is make money-handling just as simple and as systematized as you can.

FIGURE 7-2 ════════════════════════════════════

### Reimbursing Your Professional Corporation for Personal Use of Car

| | Example figures | Your figures | Line |
|---|---|---|---|
| **A.** Total mileage during tax year | 20,000 | _____ | A |
| **B.** Nonbusiness miles of use: ☐10% ☐20% ☐30% ☐40% ☐50% ☐___% | 4,000 | _____ | B |
| **C.** Rental fee payable to company for each mile of personal use | $.15 | $_____ | C |
| **D.** Rental fee to be entered as additional income on employee's W-2 statement: Line C multiplied by Line B | $600 | $_____ | D |

## Getting started in private practice

The first rule toward that end is to bank every dime received.

Whether you're practicing alone or with someone else, you need at least two checking accounts—one for the practice, one for yourself. Every dime of income from the practice needs to be banked in the practice account. All other income goes into the personal account.

Now let's make matters just a little more complicated but a whole lot smarter.

Also open a savings account for the practice. Look for the kind of savings account that pays interest from the day of deposit to the day of withdrawal. If the account is in the same bank as the practice's checking account, fine. That's a convenience.

## FIGURE 7-3

### Rental Fee Paid by Professional Corporation for Office in Home

|  |  | Example figures | Your figures | Line |
|---|---|---|---|---|
| **A.** | Purchase price of the house or apartment | $80,000 | $_____ | A |
| **B.** | Depreciation expense: Divide Line A by □45  □____ | $ 1,777 | $_____ | B |
| **C.** | Total cost of utilities for the year (gas, electricity, fuel oil, water) | $   720 | $_____ | C |
| **D.** | Total cost of services for the year (maid, lawn care, snow removal, trash removal) | $ 2,460 | $_____ | D |
| **E.** | Subtotal: Add Lines B, C, and D | $ 4,957 | $_____ | E |
| **F.** | Number of rooms in the house | 8 | _____ | F |
| **G.** | Divide Line E by Line F | $   619 | $_____ | G |
| **H.** | Purchase price of fixtures, furnishings, equipment used in office area | $ 4,200 | $_____ | H |
| **I.** | Depreciation expenses: Divide Line H by □10  □____ | $   420 | $_____ | I |
| **J.** | Annual rental fee: Add Lines G and I | $ 1,039 | $_____ | J |
| **K.** | Monthly rental fee: Line J divided by 12 | $ 86.58 | $_____ | K |

Keep a nominal amount on deposit in the checking account—say, $50—just to make sure there's always enough money there to keep the account active and to pay any charges by the bank. All the practice's receipts should be deposited in the savings account. Why? To earn interest. That interest may look small now, but in time your little solo practice may grow into a big group, and the habits you develop now may as well be the right ones.

When you sit down to sign checks written on the practice's checking account—a couple of times each month ought to get the job done—have your medical assistant write the checks, attach the bills being paid, and run an adding-machine tape on the total money to be paid out. When you put the checks in the mail, you or your assistant can transfer the same total amount from the practice's savings account to its checking account. How you do so depends on the bank or banks you're doing business with. You may need to send your assistant to the bank itself. Or you may be able to write a check on the savings account. That's commonly done these days on personal savings accounts, but it isn't often permitted with a business or professional savings account. More likely, you'll open both accounts in a commercial bank and make the transfer of funds with a phone call. That's what I do.

Now, just to complicate the banking business a little more: Also make the same dual arrangement—open a savings account and a checking account—for your personal or family money. Or open a personal savings account that lets you write checks.

Where should you bank income that's not a part of your practice? In the personal savings account. I'm thinking of money you and your spouse receive as gifts and from stock dividends or earnings from other personal investments.

How should you keep track of your practice's disbursements? First, select the right kind of checks for the job. I like to use a three-part check. The top copy pays the bill, the first carbon copy is filed by month—January, February, March—and the second carbon copy is attached to the invoice or bill paid, which is then filed in a folder by payment category. Many banks supply three-part checks on request; so does The Drawing Board, Box 505, 256 Regal Rd., Dallas, Tex. 75221.

FIGURE 7-4 ═══════════════════════════════════

## A Handy Record
## of Deductible Cash Expenses

**JOHN Q. DOKTOR, M.D.** _____/_____/19____

Mileage end of day _____

Mileage start of day _____

Mileage total _____

Personal miles:____%: _____

Gas, oil, lubrication, etc. _____

Car repairs, towing _____

Tires, battery, etc. _____

Parking, tolls, washing _____

Taxi, limousine, train, bus _____

Meeting expense: _____

    Place: _____

    Person(s): _____

    Relationship: ☐Referring doctor

    ☐Consultant ☐Patient ☐Lawyer

    ☐Accountant ☐Management consultant

    ☐ _____

    Patient or other matter discussed:

    Expenses: ☐Food, drink ☐Room ☐Steno

    ☐Audiovisual equipment rental

    ☐ _____

    ☐Receipt(s) attached ☐No receipt(s)

Postage, post office box _____

Other delivery expenses: _____

Office coffee, tea, etc. _____

Office supplies: _____

Other: _____   _____

_____   _____

_____   _____

_____   _____

    SIGNATURE: _____

Note that I mentioned invoice or bill. You may first receive an invoice from a supplier and later his bill. Or sometimes you get only the bill, no invoice. The purpose of the invoice is simply to let you know that the goods you ordered have been shipped. When the bill comes, you write your check, entering the check number on the statement and the invoice number on the check. The next month, when the canceled check comes back from the bank, staple it to the bill. Then you can file all three documents—canceled check, bill, and invoice—in a folder for the month in which you received the bank statement. Or, if your accountant suggests that you file it in the month the check was written, do that. In the view of the Internal Revenue Service, either way is fine. Just be consistent.

What's wrong with relying on check stubs? Lots. Anyone can write anything on a check stub at any time. A canceled check is much more convincing.

The month's folder should also contain the bank statement, charge slips (if used as receipts), deposit slips, daysheets (if they can be removed from the daybook), completed receipt books, and petty-cash records.

Since the words "petty cash" are not acceptable as a deduction in every T-man's eyes, you ought to be specific. When money comes out of the office cashbox, a receipt or a dated note of explanation ought to go in. When you dip into the office cash, leave your personal check for the amount taken. The check, then, will be deposited in place of the currency.

At year's end you'll have a folder full of records for each month, all neat and tidy and ready for your tax adviser's inspection. At home, you need a similar file, except this one needs to be set up by payment category, rather than by the month. The canceled-check file with monthly dividers is acceptable, but folders labeled by expense category are really better. As each bill is paid, mark the check number and the date of payment on the bill, and put it aside until the canceled check comes back; then, the canceled check can be taped or stapled to the bill paid and filed in the appropriate folder. Figure 7-1 gives you the words to put on all the labels that go on the folders.

You keep all these records virtually forever or until Congress

## Getting started in private practice

passes a law that makes it unnecessary for us to function as tax rats for the I.R.S. There's a three-year nominal requirement on keeping records for study by the I.R.S., six years when fraud is involved. But the statute on tax fraud can be extended virtually without limit. Then, too, the capital improvements to your home or condominium apartment over the entire time you own it need to be documented for tax purposes when you eventually sell. And you may need to document your defense in any future controversy with employees over their retirement-plan rights. So the nominal record-retention requirements mean nothing, really. Your best bet is simply to keep each year's records forever in a dry, safe place. Or have them microfilmed and microfiched.

Speaking of tax fraud: Watch your professional-car deduction! The tax laws do not permit any deduction for travel between your home and your first business stop of the day, but they do let you deduct for all noncommutation business-travel costs. The best deal is sometimes a terribly complicated matter to determine, and it depends on several key factors—your personal income tax bracket, the amount and percentage of practice-connected auto use, and the cost of the car. Because of the complexity, which is additionally complicated by the fact that each I.R.S. district tends to take its own

FIGURE 7-5 ═══════════════════════════════════

### Monthly Record of Production and Expenses

Use this worksheet in the first two years of your practice, right from the first month—and, of course, it doesn't need to be January just because that's the month named at the top of the form. At the end of your first month or partial month in practice, enter the various totals for that month on the form. Your year to date (YTD) totals after the second month provide the basis for a simple projection for the year; just divide by the number of months in the YTD (for example, $24,678 production divided by 6 months equals $4,113 a month), then multiply by 12 months in the year ($4,113 × 12 = $49,356). Also, enter your monthly totals for Lines A through D on the monthly tally sheet shown in Chapter 20. After 24 months, you can stop using this worksheet and move on to the more sophisticated management system in Chapter 20. The "% of A" monthly entry on this form does require a brief explanation. Just divide each month's YTD figures on Lines B through I by that month's YTD production (for example, $3,000 YTD rent divided by $24,678 YTD production equals .1215 Line E% of A).

## Monthly Record of Production and Expenses
### Year 1

| | PRODUCTION | ADJUSTMENTS: POVERTY | ADJUSTMENTS: PROFESSIONAL COURTESY | CHARGES A-B-C | OFFICE RENT | EMPLOYEE PAYROLL | OTHER BASIC OVERHEAD | TOTAL BASIC OVERHEAD E-F-G | COMPENSATION FUND D-H |
|---|---|---|---|---|---|---|---|---|---|
| | A | B | C | D | E | F | G | H | I |
| JAN-Month | | | | | | | | | |
| JAN-YTD | | | | | | | | | |
| JAN-% of A | 1.0000 | | | | | | | | |
| JAN-Projection | | | | | | | | | |
| FEB-Month | | | | | | | | | |
| FEB-YTD | | | | | | | | | |
| FEB-% of A | 1.0000 | | | | | | | | |
| FEB-Projection | | | | | | | | | |
| MAR-Month | | | | | | | | | |
| MAR-YTD | | | | | | | | | |
| MAR-% of A | 1.0000 | | | | | | | | |
| MAR-Projection | | | | | | | | | |
| APR-Month | | | | | | | | | |
| APR-YTD | | | | | | | | | |
| APR-% of A | 1.0000 | | | | | | | | |
| APR-Projection | | | | | | | | | |
| MAY-Month | | | | | | | | | |
| MAY-YTD | | | | | | | | | |
| MAY-% of A | 1.0000 | | | | | | | | |
| MAY-Projection | | | | | | | | | |
| JUN-Month | | | | | | | | | |
| JUN-YTD | | | | | | | | | |
| JUN-% | 1.0000 | | | | | | | | |

## Monthly Record of Production and Expenses
### Year 2

| | PRODUCTION | ADJUSTMENTS: POVERTY | ADJUSTMENTS: PROFESSIONAL COURTESY | CHARGES A-B-C | OFFICE RENT | EMPLOYEE PAYROLL | OTHER BASIC OVERHEAD | TOTAL BASIC OVERHEAD E-F-G | COMPENSATION FUND D-H |
|---|---|---|---|---|---|---|---|---|---|
| | A | B | C | D | E | F | G | H | I |
| JAN-Month | | | | | | | | | |
| JAN-YTD | | | | | | | | | |
| JAN-% of A | 1.0000 | | | | | | | | |
| JAN-Projection | | | | | | | | | |
| FEB-Month | | | | | | | | | |
| FEB-YTD | | | | | | | | | |
| FEB-% of A | 1.0000 | | | | | | | | |
| FEB-Projection | | | | | | | | | |
| MAR-Month | | | | | | | | | |
| MAR-YTD | | | | | | | | | |
| MAR-% of A | 1.0000 | | | | | | | | |
| MAR-Projection | | | | | | | | | |
| APR-Month | | | | | | | | | |
| APR-YTD | | | | | | | | | |
| APR-% of A | 1.0000 | | | | | | | | |
| APR-Projection | | | | | | | | | |
| MAY-Month | | | | | | | | | |
| MAY-YTD | | | | | | | | | |
| MAY-% of A | 1.0000 | | | | | | | | |
| MAY-Projection | | | | | | | | | |
| JUN-Month | | | | | | | | | |
| JUN-YTD | | | | | | | | | |
| JUN-% of A | 1.0000 | | | | | | | | |
| JUN-Proj. | | | | | | | | | |

position on deductible car expenses, there's no substitute for a good tax adviser's opinion here.

A professional corporation can own the car, take an investment tax credit and a depreciation write-off, pay the car insurance, pay for maintenance and gasoline and oil, and rent the company car to you for personal use. Figure 7-2 provides a worksheet with example figures showing all that.

The tax law also allows your professional corporation to rent office space in your home for your own use. Otherwise, the traditional home-office deduction is out the window because of the Tax Reform Act of 1976. Nonincorporated doctors who study at home or prepare lectures there are out of luck, even if they hold teaching appointments, lecture, or otherwise perform income-producing assignments requiring study and preparation at home. Until that 1976 law was passed, the I.R.S. readily accepted a deduction for a home office; the taxpayer-I.R.S. disagreements were merely about the amount of the deduction. In 1976 Congress suddenly said no deduction at all was the appropriate amount—except when a doctor conducted *all* his practice in a home-office setup completely separated from the family areas of the house. Some physicians still practice that way. They're unaffected by the new law.

However, the professional corporation's rental of the property for use by the doctor-employee who lives there is another matter, and it remains untouched by the new tax law. The money paid to the individual doctor by his corporation is a tax-deductible expense to the corporation and ordinary income to the doctor. This money is shown on his Form 1040, his personal income tax return. However, he may take offsetting deductions, including an appropriate share of the expenses of the utilities, maid service, lawn care, snow removal, and depreciation of house and furnishings. A worksheet covering all that is shown in Figure 7-3.

A third area in which the professional corporation has a special advantage is in vacation-home rental property. The Tax Reform Act of 1976 allows the owner no deduction for depreciation and maintenance expenses of such property if he uses the place more than 14 days during the year or for more than 10 per cent of its annual rental period. That 14-day limitation covers the use by any partners in ownership and by any partner's family members. The law even knocks out reciprocal deals—you stay in my condo, I'll stay in yours.

But, again, there's a corporation loophole. A corporation (though not the Subchapter S kind) may own and tax-deduct vacation rental property, even if it rents to a doctor-employee for less than a fair fee. Both individual and corporate owners can continue to take two deductions—interest and property taxes. The P.C. can then own a condominium at Vail or in Florida or wherever, put the place in the hands of a rental agent for purposes of profit, and rent it out for a pittance to vacationing doctor-employees and their families.

There is, however, a catch which could be the reason why the P.C. gets such favorable treatment. First, it must pay a corporate income tax in order to get the money to invest in the rental property. Second, some part of the money going into the property represents cash that might otherwise have been invested in each doctor-employee's retirement fund for long-term tax-free investment growth. And each $1,000 invested annually for, say, 30 years at the 15 per cent rate of growth targeted by professional investment advisers comes to $434,700—a stiff price for a supposedly cheap vacation.

So I'm not sure that the vacation condominium or the company car or any other tax gimmick that looks good at first glance is really such a good deal after all. The one tax truth that remains untarnished: That P.C. retirement plan is really all the tax break you'll ever need.

# 8

# Yes, you can
# stay out of trouble when
# selecting your office

The biggest practice-management problem you probably face right now is not having enough money to buy or lease the kind of office space and equipment you ought to have. The rough rule of thumb for office-space requirements is 1,000 square feet for each doctor in the practice, though that figure varies by specialty, productivity, and patient load. Chances are that you can afford no more than 400 to 800 square feet in your first year of practice, depending on how much per square foot you pay.

Another rule of thumb is that in a reasonably well-designed office only about 20 per cent of the total square footage can be given up to corridors, closets, toilets, and other relatively nonproductive use. So there's a good chance that you'll be faced with some hard decisions. Even in a subspecialty surgical practice, a reception room with less than 150 square feet is claustrophobic. And it's awfully hard for any practice to do with less than 150 square feet for a business office, though too many doctors try. After

FIGURE 8-1

## How Much Office Space and Equipment
## Your Practice Can Afford to Buy

| | | Example figures | Your figures | Line |
|---|---|---|---|---|
| **A.** | Production is the full value of services rendered before any adjustment. What production do you project for the practice in the next 12 months? | $165,000 | _____ | A |

**B.** Now make a list, including prices, of the clinical and business-office equipment that you'd like to acquire. Enter your items in order of priority, highest first:

1. _____ $_____
2. _____ _____
3. _____ _____
4. _____ _____
5. _____ _____
6. _____ _____
7. _____ _____
8. _____ +_____

| | | | | |
|---|---|---|---|---|
| | TOTAL: | $ 10,725 | _____ | B |

**C.** Now list your probable spending in the next 12 months for office space:

Rent (or mortgage payment) $_____
Gas, electric _____
Heat _____
Water, sewerage charge _____
Cleaning, maintenance of building _____
Snow removal, care of grounds _____
Parking _____
Other: _____ +_____

| | | | | |
|---|---|---|---|---|
| | TOTAL: | $ 9,800 | _____ | C |

| | | | | |
|---|---|---|---|---|
| **D.** | Our subjective budgeting guideline for both equipment and office space: Line A multiplied by .095 | $ 15,675 | _____ | D |
| **E.** | Your spending plan: Add Lines B and C | $ 20,525 | _____ | E |
| **F.** | If Line D is larger than Line E: Excess budget available for additional purchases: Line D minus Line E | | _____ | F |
| **G.** | Or, if Line E is larger than Line D: Amount you need to consider trimming from your equipment shopping list: Line E minus Line D | $ 4,850 | _____ | G |

allowing for both of those essential rooms, you may have space remaining for only three rooms of about 100 square feet each. One lab, one X-ray room, and one examining room? Two examining rooms and one consultation room? Or three examining rooms?

The best management answer is to go with the money rooms—the rooms that pay the rent. In most specialties, that means a vote for three examining rooms.

You can estimate your own ability to buy office space with the help of one of the worksheets accompanying this chapter. But let me give you a shortcut right here.

You'll probably have first-year production somewhere around $60,000. Whatever the figure is, don't plan on budgeting more than 8 per cent of it for office rent. If your production is $60,000, budget $4,800 a year for office rent—$400 a month. How far your budget goes depends on how fancy you feel you need to live. At a modest $4.50 a square foot annually, $4,800 buys 1,067 square feet, and that comes close to being the space you need. Around the country, the usual range for professional-office rentals is $4.50 to $8.50 a square foot. Yes, some doctors do find suitable office space for less than $4.50 a square foot, but there's no point counting on it. Space in luxury buildings easily goes as high as $20 a square foot, but it's hard to think of any big advantage in being there. Go where you can afford to be.

You'll save some money if you link forces with another doctor or two. The same minimal 300 square feet required in a solo practice for a reception room and a business office can, with careful scheduling, serve two or three doctors working in the same office. It's precisely because of such truths that almost everyone has always figured that group practice is better than solo practice.

You don't have to enter into a legal partnership with somebody to enjoy the cost-saving benefits of sharing an office. If you can find a guy who's compatible and never in the office in the mornings, you can offer to cut his office costs in half by sharing space with you if you can arrange your schedule so that you're never in the office in the afternoons.

Depending on the specialties involved, that kind of an ar-

*(Continued on page 94)*

FIGURE 8-2

## How Much Your Own Building Will Cost to Construct

| | | Example figures | Your figures | Line |
|---|---|---|---|---|
| **A.** | Number of doctors to be in the building seeing patients at any one time | 12 | _____ | A |
| **B.** | Total square feet of building based on this average per doctor: □1,225  □_____ | 14,700 | _____ | B |
| **C.** | Examining rooms per doctor based on these guidelines: □4: OB/Gyn, IM, GS, ORS □6: GP, FP, Pediatrics □8+: Geriatrics | 48 | _____ | C |
| **D.** | Approximate land requirement in square feet: Line B multiplied by 5 (1 acre is 43,500) | 73,500 | _____ | D |
| **E.** | Approximate land cost projection: Line D multiplied by □$2  □$_____ | $147,000 | _____ | E |
| **F.** | Approximate minimum number of parking spaces required: Line A multiplied by □8  □_____ | 96 | _____ | F |
| **G.** | Cost of site work, including clearing, grading, paving of parking areas, sewerage and utility connections: Line B multiplied by □$6  □_____ | $88,200 | _____ | G |
| **H.** | Organizational expenses, including topographical survey, insurance, legal and accounting fees, construction interest, engineering and development fees: Line B multiplied by □$5  □$_____ | $73,500 | _____ | H |
| **I.** | Construction cost, including carpeting, cabinets, and fixtures: Line B multiplied by □$45  □$_____ | $661,500 | _____ | I |
| **J.** | Total of land and building: Add Lines E, G, H, and I | $970,200 | _____ | J |
| **K.** | Long-term mortgage financing: Line J multiplied by □1.00 □.90 □.80 □.75 □.6667 □_____ (figure varies with availability of mortgage money; check by phoning at least one commercial mortgage department at a local bank, or project tentatively here by using □.90) · | $873,180 | _____ | K |
| **L.** | Up-front investment capital required: Line J minus Line K | $97,020 | _____ | L |
| **M.** | Multiply Line K by appropriate mortgage factor (possibly .00840854) to project monthly payment for principal and interest: | | | |

If 30-year mortgage:

| □.00699215 (7.5%) | □.00804623 (9%) | □.00840854 (9.5%) |
|---|---|---|
| □.00733765 (8%) | □.00768913 (8.5%) | □.00859154 (9.75%) | □.00877572 (10%) |

| If 25-year mortgage: | ☐.00738991 | ☐.00839196 | ☐.00873697 |
|---|---|---|---|
| | (7.5%) | (9%) | (9.5%) |
| ☐.00771816 | ☐.00805227 | ☐.00891137 | ☐.00908701 |
| (8%) | (8.5%) | (9.75%) | (10%) |

| | | | |
|---|---|---|---|
| | | $7,342.13 _____ | **M** |

**N.** Local taxes: Multiply Line B by: ☐.50 (low taxes) ☐1.50 (medium) ☐3.50 (high) ☐_____     $22,050 _____ **N**

**O.** Utilities: Multiply Line B by: ☐.60 (low rates) ☐.80 (medium) ☐1.10 (high)     $11,760 _____ **O**

**P.** Maintenance, insurance, legal and accounting fees, miscellaneous: Multiply Line B by ☐.50 (low) ☐.90 (medium) ☐1.35 (high) ☐_____     $13,230 _____ **P**

**Q.** Add Lines N, O, and P     $47,040 _____ **Q**

**R.** Multiply Line M (monthly mortgage payment) by 12 (months)     $88,105.56 _____ **R**

**S.** Total annual outlay for office space: Add Lines Q and R     $135,145.56 _____ **S**

**T.** Annual outlay per doctor: Line S divided by Line A     $11,262.13 _____ **T**

**U.** Total monthly outlay for office space: Line S (annual total) divided by 12 (months)     $11,262.13 _____ **U**

**V.** Monthly outlay per doctor: Line U divided by Line A     $938.51 _____ **V**

**W.** Minimum gross practice income required to handle that outlay (per doctor): Line T divided by 8 multiplied by 100     $140,777 _____ **W**

**X.** Gross practice income required to handle the outlay (all doctors): Line S divided by 8 multiplied by 100     $1,689,320 _____ **X**

**Y.** Gross practice income often rises 15% to 40% when a physician moves into a well-designed new office. Here, enter your current estimates of gross income per doctor for the 12 months preceding a move into a new office     $150,000 _____ **Y**

**Z.** Estimated gross practice income per doctor for the first 12 months in the new office: Line Y multiplied by: ☐1.15 (low) ☐1.25 (typical) ☐1.40 (high)     $172,500 _____ **Z**

**AA.** Considering these figures and any subjective factors that bear on the issue, can you now afford the move into a new office? Decision:     Yes, risk it ☐   Don't ☐   **AA**

**Indicate the subjective factors here:**

_____

_____

_____

_____

rangement can work just fine. The same specialty is no problem if neither of you looks on the other competitively. Mixed specialties are O.K., too, unless one is a referred-to specialty like chest surgery and the other is a referring specialty like family practice. That kind of an arrangement can be murder on the first guy, because the other referring doctors in town will be reluctant to refer patients to him, fearing that their patients will settle in at the new address with the family practitioner there.

Looking for a good space-sharing arrangement is very much worthwhile, but let's be realistic: Chances are that you'll end up equipping and laying out your own place, just as most other doctors have done before you. If so, you'll realize soon enough that you'll need to live without some of the conveniences you enjoyed in training. But if you can't send a patient down the hall for an X-ray or a test, you can, unless you're practicing somewhere remote, send him down the street or across town. Remember, doctors in solo practice only solo in a tax sense; clinically, they're in a big group practice. Solo practitioners cover for each other and freely refer patients for both diagnostic and treatment services.

If you practice out in the country, and there are some lifestyle advantages in doing so, you may have to supply some extra-cost testing facilities yourself or do without. The first of those two alternatives is obviously best, so if you're the kind who wants to head for

FIGURE 8-3 ════════════════════════════════════════

### Some Nationwide Specialists
### in Medical Office Buildings

☐ American Medical Buildings, 515 West Wells St., Milwaukee, Wis. 53203; (414) 276-2277.

☐ Marshall Erdman and Associates, Inc., 5117 University Ave., Madison, Wis. 53705; (608) 238-0211.

☐ Nationwide Medical-Dental Building Corp., 797 Market St., Oregon, Wis. 53575; (608) 835-5731.

☐ Professional Office Buildings, Inc., Doctors Park, Madison, Wis. 53705; (608) 233-0221.

the great outdoors, let yourself be recruited by one of those towns offering enough financial incentive to allow for the kind of office space and equipment you'll require.

Without the help of such financial incentives and without a good expense-sharing deal or a bundle of that family bread, you'll just have to look at your first office as a stepping-stone to the second. Choose the place and equip it with the attitude that you'll leave even the furnishings behind in a year or two or three, renting the place as it stands to someone else coming out of training and entering solo practice. That will be a good deal for him, since he'll be buying at used-equipment prices, and for you, too, since you'll then be in a position to leave all the old, inexpensive stuff behind and start from scratch with all the equipment and furnishings that you really wanted in the first place.

So keep your first-office furniture simple and functional— straight-back chairs with armrests and easy-care vinyl upholstery. Forget about soft, plush chairs and sofas; pregnant women, old people, and anyone with a bad back has a devil of a time getting out of them. For that matter, forget about sofas and benches of any kind. Most people go to the doctor's office alone, and almost everyone who does prefers to sit by himself in a chair. Put a table and table lamp in every corner of the reception room. Try to provide a closet; it doesn't have to have a door on it. And be sure that there's a foyer or some other protection from the cold between the reception room and the great outdoors.

The reception desk needs to be in the business office, since the reception secretary will undoubtedly be doing other kinds of work, too. And, one way or another, what she says on the phone should not be audible to people in the reception room. All conversations with patients, even including patients' identities, should be treated as confidential information by everyone in the office. That's basic medical ethics. So a secretarial desk plopped down at the end of an open reception room just won't do. You need a separate business office and a sliding glass window to separate it from the reception room.

Interior walls separating consultation rooms may need to be insulated to ensure conversational privacy between doctor and patient. Music, kept at a very low volume, can help there, and so can carpeting throughout the office. Carpeting also helps cut down on drafts, as do storm windows and heavy draperies. A thermostat in every office is ideal; two-zone heating and air-conditioning is minimal—one thermostat in the reception room, another for the rest of the office. These days, many people like a temperature of about 68 degrees, which is just fine for the reception room in most practices. The examining rooms need to be a bit warmer, since patients will be in various stages of undress. Elderly patients need warmer temperatures than the young and middle-aged.

You may have to pay for partitioning, carpeting, and the like yourself. Landlords generally don't like to pay such costs. These are leasehold improvements, and they're generally considered the tenant's responsibility. That's not to say that it's impossible to talk a landlord into paying for the improvements; to get a tenant, particularly a tenant he especially wants, he may feel that he needs to make such a concession, putting up his own capital. Chances are, though, that he'll pass along the costs to you in higher rent.

You've probably heard that there's no such thing as a standard lease, and that's true. You needn't accept a printed lease. Landlords like to make potential tenants think that leases are standard and thus mandatory because printed leases are invariably landlords' leases. Your best protection is a review of any lease, whether printed or typed, by a lawyer or a medical management consultant or both. Either kind of expert can demand that the landlord amend the lease so that he's required to install or put into good working order the following: electrical service, toilet facilities, plumbing, heating and air-conditioning units, an entryway or foyer, corridor, steps or an elevator, cracked or broken windows.

Your adviser can also make sure that you've got the right to make such corrections yourself and to deduct the cost of them from the rent if the landlord doesn't come through. After all, the person you deal with when you negotiate a lease may not be the person you deal with later. The first person may be only the landlord's agent, and he may be replaced by another. And the property, including your lease, may be sold to a new owner who lives far away, possibly even in another country.

Also, your adviser may renegotiate certain terms dealing with the leasehold improvements. A landlord's lease usually requires a tenant to remove all alterations, additions, and improvements in a careful and workmanlike manner, even though such a requirement isn't always in the interest of the landlord or the tenant. It's better to have the lease amended so that you don't need to remove any specific improvements that the landlord agrees can be left on your departure—new walls, for example. Remember: The landlord when you leave the place may not be the landlord you deal with at the start, and there's no telling what kind of a person the new owner may be. So you don't dare sign an agreement and amend it orally; put everything in writing.

Despite what some landlord or rental agent may tell you, printed leases are amended at least four times out of every five. One common addition required by medical management consultants is a paragraph freeing a doctor-tenant or his heirs from all leasehold obligations four to six months after a doctor's death or total disability. When faced with an obstinate landlord, consultants are sometimes willing to compromise by getting an option to sublet.

They also try to avoid leases with cost-of-living clauses. Virtually all commercial mortgages in most parts of the country are written so that the landlord's interest expense—often his greatest single expanse—is locked in, regardless of subsequent changes in the cost of living. So a cost-of-living clause can be hard for a landlord to defend; it's usually just a gimmick to increase his profits. A tax-escalation clause, however, is quite another matter. No one knows what's going to happen to taxes on a piece of property, but changes generally range from a little higher to a lot higher. It's fair to accept your prorated share of any tax increase on the building.

Management consultants often push for the doctor's right to renew the lease under the same terms and conditions—for instance, the right to renew a three-year lease under the same terms for two successive three-year periods.

And consultants generally try to get a printed lease's requirement that a tenant give six months' advance notice of renewal turned around so that the burden of memory is on the landlord. The clause can be amended so that renewal is automatic if you

**97**

don't move out. Or, if the landlord insists on notice of intent, an amendment can place the burden of questioning your intent on him. The idea is simply to keep you from being penalized for forgetfulness.

Some management consultants prefer to amend any clause requiring the landlord to redecorate. They recognize that a doctor's taste may be considerably different from the landlord's. A favorite way to amend that clause is to provide for a credit—some specific sum of money to be withheld from the rent at some specific future time—to be used as reimbursement to the doctor-tenant for any redecorating that is arranged for and supervised by him.

Parking and cleaning are two other matters of concern. You'll need a parking space for each doctor, present and future, plus adequate parking for employees and patients. Almost any solo practice requires a minimum of eight spaces. Cleaning services are best arranged for and paid for by the tenant, except possibly for common areas like exterior corridors in a multitenant building. Inside your own suite you'll have better control over the quality of cleaning service if you, rather than the landlord, sign the checks. Removing such a burden of payment from the landlord's wallet is grounds for an appropriate reduction in rent.

After you're established in practice and have a good fix on your projected production and income, your best deal on office space may very well be to own your own. Since that's very likely some distance down the road for you, there's no point wasting your time discussing the ins and outs of building ownership with you here. But to satisfy your curiosity as to the investment and the kind of figuring needed for your own building, I've included in this chapter a worksheet that can help you estimate, with reasonable accuracy, the price of building your own office (see Figure 8-2).

# 9

## Some of the best financial management friends you'll ever have: The medical cataloguers

Fred Maguire, a friend who was my adviser at Ohio State long ago, once told me about the time he was called into his boss's office and handed the assignment of running the annual endowed lecture. The job mainly involved hiring some big-shot newspaper columnist or editor or publisher or some TV anchorman to come to Columbus and deliver a one-hour speech on the state of the Fourth Estate— before an empty auditorium. Well, almost empty. The journalism faculty members would always show up, as would any of their students who were worried about making grades good enough to stay in school through the football season.

"Some job you've got now, Maguire," a faculty-buddy muttered sympathetically to Fred.

"Piece of cake," replied Maguire. "Just watch. I'll fill the joint with bodies."

"You're kidding. How?"

"I'll start charging admission."

**99**

He charged $3.50 a seat to attend a lecture that for years had been free, and he *did* fill the joint—that year and every year afterward until, much to his department head's dismay, he retired.

Professor Maguire's experience flashes across my mind every time I see a throwaway publication of unusual quality. I use the word "throwaway" because your older colleagues love to call all sorts of super publications by that name, and they mean it to be disparaging. But just because a magazine's free doesn't mean it's worthless.

FIGURE 9-1 ═══════════════════════════════════════

## A Sampling of Medical Cataloguers, Printers, and Business Systems

☐ Associated Business Systems, Box 1166, 512 Fourth St. South, Great Falls, Mont. 59403.

☐ Bibbero Systems, Inc., 36 Second St., San Francisco, Calif. 94105.

☐ Black & Skaggs Associates, Box 1130, 1201 Security National Bank Bldg., Battle Creek, Mich. 49016.

☐ Business Envelope Manufacturers, Inc., 615 East Broadway, Anaheim, Calif. 92805; Box 210, Melrose Park, Ill. 60160; 2350 Lafayette Ave., Bronx, N.Y. 10473; Cullom Street, Clinton, Tenn. 37716.

☐ The Colwell Company, 201 Kenyon Rd., Champaign, Ill. 61820.

☐ Control-o-Fax/Creative Systems, Inc., Box 778, 3070 West Airline Hwy., Waterloo, Iowa 50704.

☐ Cyril-Scott Company, Box 310, Lancaster, Ohio 43130.

☐ The Drawing Board, Inc., Box 505, 256 Regal Rd., Dallas, Tex. 75221.

☐ Health Management Systems, 1455 Broad St., Bloomfield, N.J. 07033.

☐ Histacount Corp., Walt Whitman Rd., Melville, N.Y. 11746.

☐ McBee Systems, 600 Washington Ave., Carlstadt, N.J. 07072.

☐ Medical Arts Press, 2900 Aldrich Ave. South, Minneapolis, Minn. 55408.

☐ New England Business Service, Inc., Townsend, Mass. 01469.

☐ Patient Care Systems, Inc., Box 1245, Darien, Conn. 06820.

☐ Physicians Record Co., 3000 South Ridgeland Ave., Berwyn, Ill. 60402.

☐ Safeguard Business Systems, 470 Maryland Dr., Fort Washington, Pa. 19034.

☐ Shingles, Inc., Box 429, Wayzata, Minn. 55391.

# FIGURE 9-2

## The Superbill

This multipurpose charge slip or superbill is designed to provide information required by insurers for reimbursement of patient services, but it can be used for all in-office patients. An assistant enters the patient's name and previous balance; the doctor circles the services rendered, enters a diagnosis, and indicates the time and duration of the next appointment. The patient is asked to give the slip to the financial secretary, who enters the fee information, strikes a total balance due, and asks, "Would you like to pay by cash or by check?" The slip also serves as a receipt and an appointment reminder. To obtain reimbursement, the patient attaches his copy of the slip to his insurance form after filling in the top part of that form (the identity section) and then submits the form and slip directly to the carrier. If you provide few or no insured services in your office, you needn't buy superbill charge slips. Cataloguers offer a variety of less comprehensive slips. Just look over the offerings and select the version that seems to suit your practice best.

John Q. Doktor, M.D.
123 Main St.
Anytown, U.S.A. 07666

**09829**

For appointment: (201) 555-1234
Billing inquiries: (201) 555-1235

Insurance inquiries: (201) 555-1236
All other matters: (201) 555-1233

ACCOUNT Jane Smith
ACCOUNT ADDRESS 321 Main St.
DATE 6-20-78
PATIENT'S NAME Susan

| SERVICE | FEE | SERVICE | FEE |
|---|---|---|---|
| Initial visit to office: | | Laboratory testing: | |
| Brief visit | 90000 | Bilirubin | 82250/90 |
| Limited visit | 90010 | Calcium, blood | 82310/90 |
| Intermediate visit | 90015 | Potassium | 84132/90 |
| Comprehensive visit | 90020 | Sodium | 84295/90 |
| Follow-up visit: | | PBI | 83533/90 |
| Minimal service | 90030 | T3 | 83539/90 |
| Limited service | 90050 | Urinalysis, micro. | 81015 |
| Intermediate service | 90060 | VDRL PM PN RT TC | 96592 |
| Comprehensive service | 90080 | | |

THIS SECTION TO BE COMPLETED FOR MEDICARE
☑ OFFICE   ☐ HOSPITAL   ☐ NURSING HOME   ☐ HOME   ☐ ____
CMT DIAG. # 4047
DOCTOR'S SIGNATURE John Q. Doktor , M.D.

MAKE NOTE OF YOUR NEXT APPOINTMENT
MONTH June   DAY 27
TIME 9:00   AM
PLEASE CALL AT LEAST 24 HOURS IN ADVANCE
FOR ANY CHANGE IN YOUR APPOINTMENT.
BRING: Urine Specimen

OFFICE USE ONLY
M. / TU / W. / TH. / F.
1 WEEKS ____MONTHS
☑ A.M.   ☐ P.M.   ☐ ____

THIS IS YOUR RECEIPT

PAID BY   ☐ CURRENCY
          ☑ CHECK
          ☐ M. O.
          ☐ ____

PREVIOUS BALANCE   $ 18
TODAY'S FEE   + 21
TODAY'S BALANCE DUE $ 39
TODAY'S PAYMENT – 25
BALANCE DUE, IF ANY $ 14

I feel much the same way about the free catalogues you'll be receiving from the various medical stationers. They arrive free because those people want and need your business, not because the products they offer are no good. For your purposes, in fact, the goods offered in their catalogues are more to the point of your needs than most of the stuff you'll see in your neighborhood office-supplies store. That place has something for everyone; the medical cataloguer has nothing but timesaving, worksaving equipment and forms and other things of value for medical offices.

Catalogues are constantly updated, with new and improved offerings being added to time-tested old favorites, so I'll do no more here than give you a sampling of what you can expect to find. Naturally, any prices I mention in this chapter or elsewhere will probably have changed by the time the words are in front of you. I mention prices simply to give you some rough idea of what you may have to pay.

1. *Money-makers.* Any doctor who sees a particular patient on a regular basis—every two months or so, or every year—can either rely on the patient's memory, or ask the patient if he'd like to receive a reminder about when to come in again. When given the choice, most patients ask for the reminder.

Filling such a request is a perfectly ethical way to recall

FIGURE 9-3 ═══════════════════════════════════════════════════

### The Daysheet

Working from data previously entered on the charge slip, an assistant enters the key financial information for each patient seen on a daysheet like this. She also enters each payment that arrives by mail—either on the same daysheet or on a second page, which can be attached to the first at day's end. Totals are struck daily, and the bank-deposit slip's total should match that of the payment column. The assistant who runs the day's adding machine tape should sign the tape and attach it to the daysheet. The assistant who fills in the bank-deposit slip should do the same—attaching either the original or a copy, as your accountant wishes. Coding is provided here to make it easy to track the various kinds of adjustments, first daily, then monthly. All adjustments fall into two categories—courtesy (friends, relatives, other doctors, Blue Shield) and poverty (Medicaid, Medicare, others).

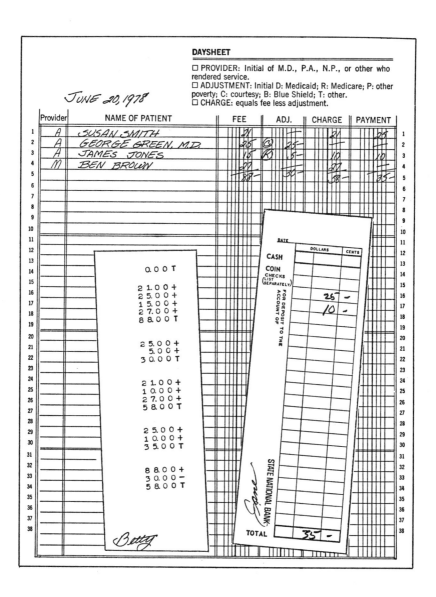

**DAYSHEET**

JUNE 20, 1978

☐ PROVIDER: Initial of M.D., P.A., N.P., or other who rendered service.
☐ ADJUSTMENT: Initial D: Medicaid; R: Medicare; P: other poverty; C: courtesy; B: Blue Shield; T: other.
☐ CHARGE: equals fee less adjustment.

| Provider | NAME OF PATIENT | FEE | ADJ. | CHARGE | PAYMENT |
|---|---|---|---|---|---|
| A | SUSAN SMITH | 21 | | 21 | 25 |
| A | GEORGE GREEN, M.D. | 25 | © 25 | | 25 |
| A | JAMES JONES | 15 | ® 5 | 10 | 10 |
| M | BEN BROWN | 27 | | 27 | |
| | | 88 | 30 | 58 | 35 |

0.00 T
21.00 +
25.00 +
15.00 +
27.00 +
88.00 T

25.00 +
5.00 +
30.00 T

21.00 +
10.00 +
27.00 +
58.00 T

25.00 +
10.00 +
35.00 T

88.00 +
30.00 −
58.00 T

Betty

DATE

| | DOLLARS | CENTS |
|---|---|---|
| CASH | | |
| COIN | | |
| CHECKS (LIST SEPARATELY) | | |
| | 25 | − |
| | 10 | − |

FOR DEPOSIT TO THE ACCOUNT OF

STATE NATIONAL BANK

| TOTAL | 35 | − |

FIGURE 9-4 ═══════════════════════════════════════

## Controlling the Office Cash

It's no problem keeping the accounts receivable updated if you keep score daily. The same goes for the change fund and the office petty cash. Some of the daysheets sold by the medical cataloguers come with updating guides something like these imprinted on the sheet. Just be sure your staff members fill in the blanks daily; it's a chore that's often skipped in badly run offices. The accounts receivable total tells you how much money is likely to be collected, minus a few percentage points for noncollectible accounts. Thus, an account that's turned over to a collector should, like a payment, reduce your accounts receivable.

### Accounts Receivable

| | | |
|---|---|---|
| Yesterday | $ | _____ |
| Today | $ | _____ |
| Charges | + | _____ |
| Payments | − | _____ |
| Subtotal | | _____ |
| To collector | − | _____ |
| End of day | | _____ |

### Change Fund

| | | |
|---|---|---|
| Yesterday | $ | _____ |
| Today | $ | _____ |
| Explanation of any difference: | | _____ |

_____

_____

### Petty Cash

| | | |
|---|---|---|
| Yesterday | $ | _____ |
| Today | $ | _____ |
| Paid out | − | _____ |
| Added | + | _____ |
| End of day | | _____ |
| Do receipts total same amount paid out? | ☐YES | ☐NO |
| If not, why? | _____ | |

_____

_____

patients for services, such as comprehensive annual physical exams. Medical Arts Press offers a selection of ethically correct recall messages for under 2 cents each in lots of 1,000. Or, if you prefer your own wording, they'll print them your way for an extra $4.

2. *Billing and collection aids.* The superbill, which we'll discuss in Chapter 11, is available in its most comprehensive version from Bibbero Systems; it costs $0.0584 each in lots of 10,000, including custom imprinting. Other charge slips, also excellent, are available from the same source for as little as $0.027 each.

No single device can head off misunderstandings over fees, billing procedures, and insurance matters the way an office-policy leaflet can. Medical Arts Press will print up your own customized version for as little as 4½ cents each.

If you expect to send a bill to someone, you'd better have the correct name and address of the responsible party and some other information, too, such as his medical-insurance policy numbers and the names of his employer and next of kin. You get all that and more with the help of a patient registration system, such as one offered by Bibbero Systems for as little as $0.0215 a form.

Standard health-insurance claim forms help your insurance secretary zip through her working day, and they're widely available. For example, there's a two-part, carbonless version for $0.028 each from the order department of the American Medical Association. (Write for a copy of the A.M.A. publication list.)

Bibbero Systems offers a standardized, six-part workmen's compensation form for less than 11 cents each in lots of 500.

Forms for collecting information on Medicare patients are available from Medical Arts Press for $0.264 each in lots of 1,000.

There's nothing like a printed message to speed the communications required to straighten out insurance-claims problems; you can get an excellent selection from Bibbero Systems, Medical Arts Press, and Colwell.

The best payment-reminder notices offered, in my opinion, are available in pads of 50—with a big selection of time-tested messages in appropriate sequence—from Bibbero Systems; the cost is $1.45 for each pad. In addition to this, a manual that spells out collection policies, procedures, and timetables is available at no charge when you place a collection-pad order of $10 or more.

    3. *Overhead management.* Colwell offers a fine inventory-control system for $13.60.

    Just about everybody offers good accounts-payable systems, but my favorite is the three-part check sold by The Drawing Board; 1,000 checks cost $48.25.

    4. *Time management.* I think the best appointment books are those offered by Bibbero Systems; an appointment book with dividers and the first year's pages costs $21.65; refill pages for the second year cost $14.70.

    On the other hand, Colwell will send you a free kit that enables you to custom-design your own appointment book, which it will then print for a fee to be quoted after the company takes a look at what you've designed.

    Colwell also offers a surgery log for $5.95.

    Both Bibbero Systems and Colwell offer patient history questionnaires; you need to look at both kinds before ordering; content, rather than price, is the deciding factor here.

    Among the relatively minor but nonetheless useful, timesaving items are Colwell's phone-message slips, the Medical Arts Press

*(Continued on page 112)*

FIGURE 9-5 ════════════════════════════════════

## Daily Totals

The daily totals for production, adjustments, charges, and payments can be entered on a form like this. Your assistant can make copies by running a master through your photocopier or a photocopier at your hospital or county medical society. By keeping an orderly record of the various daily totals, she can easily tally the month's total with the help of an adding machine. But you don't need to invent your own charge slips, daysheets, or other basic bookkeeping forms; they're sold by all the medical cataloguers. You need only select from their offerings. Their names and addresses appear in Figure 9-1.

YTD and LST 12, at the bottom of this form, mean year to date and last 12 months. Each new month's total is added to the previous month's YTD to give you this month's YTD. For a new LST 12 total, first enter last month's LST 12 figure; then add this month's monthly total; finally, subtract the monthly total for the same month last year, working from last year's totaling sheet (not shown).

DAILY TOTALS

☑ Total practice
☐ Dr. _____
☐

☐ Production (fees)  ☐ Adjustments (poverty)
☐ Adjustments (courtesy)  ☐ Charges  ☑ Payments
☐

YEAR: _____

| | JAN | FEB | MAR | APR | MAY | JUN | JUL | AUG | SEP | OCT | NOV | DEC |
|---|---|---|---|---|---|---|---|---|---|---|---|---|
| 1 | | 1,954 | 2,2 | | 1,812 | 980 | | | | | | |
| 2 | | | 0.00 T | | 1,644 | 1,101 | | | | | | |
| 3 | | 2 0.7 8 1.0 0 + | | 459 | 1,933 | | | | | | | |
| 4 | | 6 4.0 3 3.0 0 + | | 216 | 890 | | | | | | | |
| 5 | | 8 4.8 1 4.0 0 T | | 040 | 111 | 965 | | | | | | |
| 6 | | 1 7 5.5 3 6.0 0 + | | | | 119 | | | | | | |
| 7 | | 2 0.7 8 1.0 0 + | | | | 72 | | | | | | |
| 8 | | 1 7.3 2 1.0 0 – | | | | 79 | | | | | | |
| 9 | | 1 7 8.9 9 6.0 0 T | | | | 38 | | | | | | |
| 10 | | | | | | | | | | | | |
| 11 | | | | | | | | | | | | |
| 12 | .37 | | 1.8 1 2.0 0 + | | | 44 | | | | | | |
| 13 | 42 | | 1.6 4 4.0 0 + | | | 40 | | | | | | |
| 14 | | | 1.9 3 3.0 0 + | | | 30 | | | | | | |
| 15 | | | 8 9 0.0 0 + | | 76 | 118 | | | | | | |
| 16 | .33 | | 1 1 1.0 0 + | | 0 | 220 | | | | | | |
| 17 | 4.5 | | 3 9 5.0 0 + | | | | | | | | | |
| 18 | 80 | | 3 7 7.0 0 + | | 88 | | | | | | | |
| 19 | 60 | | 3 6 7.0 0 + | | 5 | | | | | | | |
| 20 | 29 | | 3 5 7.0 0 + | | 78 | 62 | | | | | | |
| 21 | | | 5 0 0.0 0 + | | | 35 | | | | | | |
| 22 | | | 3 9 6.0 0 + | | | | | | | | | |
| 23 | .37 | | 3 8 0.0 0 + | | 70 | | | | | | | |
| 24 | 161 | | 3 8 8.0 0 + | | 171 | | | | | | | |
| 25 | 1,642 | | 7 5.0 0 + | | 00 | 39 | | | | | | |
| 26 | 1,850 | | 8 8.0 0 + | | | 543 | | | | | | |
| 27 | 1,525 | | 3 7 0.0 0 + | | | | | | | | | |
| 28 | | 1,912 | 2,102 | 2,630 | | | | | | | | |
| 29 | | 1,972 | | | 2,270 | | | | | | | |
| 30 | 1,605 | | 4,855 | | 1,465 | | | | | | | |
| 31 | 1,782 | | 3,180 | | 1,510 | | | | | | | |
| Mo. | 15,594 | 9,462 | 18,373 | 20,604 | 20,781 | | | | | | | |
| YTD | 15,594 | 25,056 | 43,429 | 64,033 | 84,814 | | | | | | | |
| LST 12 | 168,382 | 169,321 | 172,458 | 175,536 | 178,996 | | | | | | | |

Within inset slip (partial column of entries):
3 9 5.0 0 +
3 7 7.0 0 +
3 6 7.0 0 +
3 5 7.0 0 +
5 0 0.0 0 +
3 9 6.0 0 +
3 8 0.0 0 +
3 8 8.0 0 +
7 5.0 0 +
8 8.0 0 +
3 7 0.0 0 +
4 7 1.0 0 +
7 0 0.0 0 +
1.7 3 9.0 0 +
2.5 4 3.0 0 +
2.2 7 0.0 0 +
1.4 6 5.0 0 +
1.5 1 0.0 0 +
2 0.7 8 1.0 0 T

FIGURE 9-6

## Monthly Totals

Monthly totals can then be entered on another form of your own making—something about like this one.

**MONTHLY TOTALS**
☑ Total practice
☐ Dr. _____
☐ _____

| Month | PRODUCTION (Fee) | ADJ. Total | ADJ. D,R,P | ADJ. C | ADJ. B,T | CHARGE (Net) | RECEIPTS (Pay) |
|---|---|---|---|---|---|---|---|
| 1978 | 17,745 | 200 | 80 | 25 | 125 | 17,465 | 15,598 |
| FEB | 11,504 | 150 | 50 | 15 | 85 | 11,354 | 9,962 |
| MAR | 20,539 | 145 | 45 | 25 | 75 | 20,394 | 18,323 |
| APR | 23,560 | 210 | 110 | 35 | 65 | 23,350 | 20,609 |
| MAY | 27,280 | 265 | 90 | 65 | 110 | 27,015 | 24,791 |
| JUN | | | | | | | |
| JUL | | | | | | | |
| AUG | | | | | | | |
| SEP | | | | | | | |
| OCT | | | | | | | |
| NOV | | | | | | | |
| DEC | | | | | | | |
| 19 | | | | | | | |
| FEB | | | | | | | |
| MAR | | | | | | | |
| APR | | | | | | | |
| MAY | | | | | | | |
| JUN | | | | | | | |
| JUL | | | | | | | |
| AUG | | | | | | | |
| SEP | | | | | | | |
| OCT | | | | | | | |
| NOV | | | | | | | |
| DEC | | | | | | | |
| 19 | | | | | | | |
| FEB | | | | | | | |
| MAR | | | | | | | |
| APR | | | | | | | |
| MAY | | | | | | | |
| JUN | | | | | | | |
| JUL | | | | | | | |
| AUG | | | | | | | |
| SEP | | | | | | | |
| OCT | | | | | | | |
| NOV | | | | | | | |
| DEC | | | | | | | |

NOTES: ☐ PRODUCTION is the value of services rendered (full, unadjusted fee). ☐ D: Medicaid ☐ R: Medicare ☐ P: other poverty reduction ☐ C: courtesy ☐ B: Blue Shield ☐ T: other adjustment ☐ CHARGE: net fee after adjustment from full fee. ☐ RECEIPTS: payment for services rendered, whether by cash, check, or money order and whether by patient or third party.

FIGURES 9-7 and 9-8

## Totals for Adjustments

Alternatively, the adjustments can be tallied in greater detail, both daily and monthly. At first, the purpose may be no more than informational. In time, though, you may see worrisome trends developing that may lead you to a decision—to drop Blue Shield participation, for instance, or to extend professional courtesy to fewer persons. Longer range, a public relations problem may be lessened in the event of an attack on you for seemingly accepting too much in Medicaid, Medicare, or other public funds. The many doctors who have been subjected to public criticism by Federal and state agency reports to the press have generally had no countering figures in hand—for example, the amount of services given away in adjustments to Medicaid patients, which is the kind of information a local newspaper may easily recognize as an appropriate part of the story. Such totals are becoming significant to doctors who continue to accept Medicaid patients.

**DAILY TOTALS FOR ADJUSTMENTS**

☑ Total practice
☐ Dr. _____
☐ _____

| | | D | R | P | C | B | T | | |
|---|---|---|---|---|---|---|---|---|---|
| Mo.4/78 | TOTAL | Medicaid | Medicare | Other poverty | Courtesy | Blues | Other | | |
| 1 | 12 | 5 | | | | 7 | | | |
| 2 | 8 | 3 | | | | 5 | | | |
| 3 | | | | | | | | | |
| 4 | | | | | | | | | |
| 5 | 10 | | | | | 10 | | | |
| 6 | 0 | | | | | | | | |
| 7 | 0 | | | | | | | | |
| 8 | 10 | 5 | | | | 5 | | | |
| 9 | 0 | | | | | | | | |
| 10 | | | | | | | | | |
| 11 | | | | | | | | | |
| 12 | 10 | | 10 | | | | | | |
| 13 | 25 | | 10 | | | 5 | 10 Staff | | |
| | 20 | 5 | 5 | | | 10 | | | |
| 30 | | | | | | | | | |
| 31 | | | | | | | | | |
| MONTH | | | | | | | | | |
| YTD | | | | | | | | | |
| LAST 12 | | | | | | | | | |

**MONTHLY TOTALS FOR ADJUSTMENTS**

☑ Total practice
☐ Dr. _____
☐ _____

| | | D | R | P | C | B | T | | |
|---|---|---|---|---|---|---|---|---|---|
| 19 78 | TOTAL | Medicaid | Medicare | Other poverty | Courtesy | Blues | Other | | |
| JAN | 280 | 50 | 30 | — | 25 | 175 | — | | |
| FEB | 150 | 10 | 40 | — | 15 | 50 | 35 — Staff | | |
| MAR | 175 | 35 | 10 | — | 25 | 70 | 5 — Staff | | |
| APR | 210 | 80 | 30 | — | 35 | 50 | 15 — Cash Missing | | |
| MAY | 265 | 70 | 20 | — | 65 | 65 | 45 — Staff | | |
| JUN | | | | | | | | | |
| JUL | | | | | | | | | |
| AUG | | | | | | | | | |
| SEP | | | | | | | | | |

FIGURE 9-9

## Out-of-Office Charge Slip

Some medical cataloguers offer out-of-office charge slips something like this one. It helps keep tabs on services that some doctors often forget—and thus never record, bill, or get paid for. Always avoid any "system" that depends on memory.

This three-by-five card slips easily into a shirt pocket. An assistant fills in the identification side. On the other side, the doctor circles the appropriate printed service code or writes in the code (if he remembers it) or the descriptive words themselves (if he doesn't) if the service is not printed on the card. If an assistant accompanies him to the hospital, she may see that the cards get back to the financial secretary. Otherwise, the doctor returns them.

Front

Back

FIGURE 9-10

## Ledger Card

Before buying a supply of ledger cards, select your billing method (see Chapter 11). Most computer-billing systems bypass the ledger card; an equivalent is printed by the computer. Shingled-billing systems come with a ledger card. You need to buy cards for any record-keeping system that includes photocopy billing.

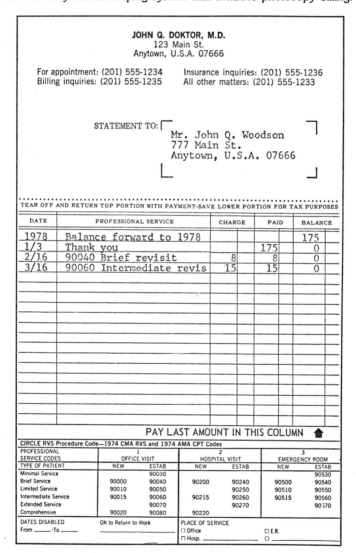

examining-room signal system, Bibbero System's filing labels and signal dots, Drawing Board's self-inking rubber stamps (including a signature stamp), and Histacount's paper-stamp affixing gadget, called Stamp E-Z.

5. *Clinical records.* Colwell's data-imprinted medical records jacket is a favorite among many doctors; 1,000 for $94.

And chart secretaries everywhere are enthusiastic about pressure-sensitive transcribing paper, available in 7-inch widths from Associated Business Systems and in 8-inch widths from Medical Arts Press.

6. *Personnel forms and records.* Bibbero is clearly the leader here, in my view, with a comprehensive hiring system for just $10.60—one pad (25 forms) of job-application forms specifically designed for medical-office employment, another pad of interview evaluation forms, a pad of personnel records (one for each employee), and complete instructions in a booklet entitled "The Doctor's Hiring Manual."

In the next chapter, we'll take up what you can order by mail to set fair fees. Now, tell me: If you can get something free to help you do that, will you bother to order it? If not, maybe I can make special arrangements for you to get it through Professor Maguire, who will make you pay $3.50 for it so that you'll love it.

# 10

## Best practice management advice you'll ever get: How to set your fees

The most sensible way I know for physicians to set fees is to use the relative value study—California's. It's rationally based, a result of many years of study, debate, and compromise by a multispecialty committee. Key state societies have recommended it for their members' use. About half the physicians in private practice in this country are in states that have adopted the California Relative Value Studies (C.R.V.S.) as their own. I recommend it to you highly if you can get hold of a copy.

The problem is that the Federal Trade Commission, which rightfully concerns itself with conspiracies within any industry to fix prices to the detriment of consumers, is against the C.R.V.S. approach or, at least, against some variations of that approach. It has directed certain specialty societies to stop publishing, stop distributing, and otherwise to stop using relative values of their own design, possibly because of the single-specialty use. As I write these words, no such directive has come from the F.T.C. to the California

**113**

Medical Association or to any of the state societies that have adopted the C.R.V.S.

Any such order would be a shame. The C.R.V.S. is *not* a fee schedule. It's a study, a report, a weighing of each service against others expressed in units or points. Underlying it are all kinds of cross-specialty considerations, including skill, dexterity, and length of training required for competence in given procedures. It's up to the individual doctor to say how many dollars each point is worth and, through multiplication, to determine his own fee schedule. The C.R.V.S. is simply a tool designed to help the practitioner set *fair* fees and to help patients and consumer organizations determine if a practitioner's fees are, in fact, fair.

From the start, the C.R.V.S. has been widely accepted by Medicare carriers and by the Department of Health, Education and Welfare administrators overseeing the Medicare program. When Medicare came into being, the most likely alternative to the C.R.V.S. was the Blue Shield fee schedule, but H.E.W. quickly saw that the Blue Shield schedule made no sense at all.

Blue Shield's approach was to determine the fees actually charged by doctors and, from that information, more or less average out the figures and thus create fee schedules. Logical? Well, there wasn't much logic in doctors' fees to begin with. The first practitioner in a community would pick fees out of the air, and later arrivals would do the same or charge what the first physician charged. Result? Wild differences from one community to the next, as you'd anticipate. Until the C.R.V.S. came along, no serious, rational, interdisciplinary study was made of fair values of physicians' services. All Blue Shield did was add up lots of nonsense figures and then average them out.

I can't believe that the F.T.C. actually wants private practitioners to go back to setting fees by guess and by gosh, and I can't believe that H.E.W. will stand still for the F.T.C.'s removal of a tool that has served doctors, consumers, and Government well. But it could happen, so I suggest that you order a C.R.V.S. manual directly from the California Medical Association. If you find that the F.T.C. has closed down deliveries, write a letter of protest to your Congressman and both Senators and to H.E.W. Any such decision would be silly, and all those people need to be told as much—by you, not just by me.

The C.R.V.S. manual includes a detailed explanation and covers all kinds of exceptions and instructions. I won't bother trying to cover any of that here. It all becomes understandable with the manual in your hands.

And there's little that it doesn't cover—except for fee-setting pointers like these:

● *Control your time.* The C.R.V.S. manual rightfully points out that a fair fee for a brief visit is a fraction of that for a full visit, but it doesn't remind you that the length of a visit can depend more on you than on a patient's needs.

Your job is to diagnose and to treat. You can delegate to trained medical assistants the task of gathering information through labwork, diagnostic X-rays, initial histories, and the like.

If you must waste a patient's time chatting about fishing or the Big Game or the weather, do it on your own nickel.

● *Itemize every service rendered.* That's the fairest way.

The C.R.V.S. manual helps you to identify the services you perform in your practice and to establish a fair fee for each, but the manual can't help you remember to indicate every service performed. Charge slips help you do that. Use them.

If you charge an appropriate fee for every injection, every overtime counseling session, and every other extra-cost service, you'll feel less pressure to raise fees across the board or to raise your basic office-visit fee. When you raise that fee, you make the patients who come in for routine visits help pay for the extraordinary services. What's fair about that?

● *Control your phone time.* O.K., so the telephone isn't a big problem in all specialties. But it sure is in some.

Pediatrics is the obvious example. Many pediatricians have established a morning phone-in hour, often the first office hour of the day. That arrangement has helped keep many a pediatrician's phone quiet at night. A mother with a sick kid will often not bother the doctor during the sleeping hours when she feels assured of getting through to him first thing in the morning.

By and large, your older colleagues do not charge for phone

advice—not even in pediatrics. Most medical management consultants advise physicians not to.

● *Never charge interest for slow payment.* In the view of the American Medical Association's Judicial Council, charging interest is just plain unethical.

On the other hand, I've never heard anyone say it's unethical to give a discount for payment at the time of service, and some management people I know do advise giving such a discount to help encourage patients to pay then. After all, bookkeeping and billing costs are saved.

Try putting this printed notice near the financial secretary's window or desk: "Because of the savings in accounting and billing costs, a 5 per cent reduction in fees will accompany payment at the time of service." Such wording is less offensive than the more widely seen notice: "Please pay at the time of service."

● *Be careful how much you give away in professional courtesy.* If you ask your colleagues or the executive director of your county medical society, you'll probably hear that the tendency in your area is for doctors to buy health insurance, often through a group Blue Cross-Blue Shield plan arranged by the society. Therefore, another doctor who looks after a member of the insured doctor's family should receive the insured portion of his regular fee. Just have your financial secretary ask if the doctor's family has health insurance before she charges off the visit to professional courtesy.

I do hope that you won't forget to order a copy of the California Relative Value Studies manual. Your state society's headquarters may offer its version of the California manual, or may distribute the C.R.V.S., possibly in its own name. One of your colleagues may have a copy that he's willing to lend you. Or your medical management consultant may have one. If he doesn't, he can get a copy.

# 11

# Billing and collecting: Getting paid in full and on time

Time was when a doctor who'd accept a credit card in payment of his bill was castigated by his peers. In the late 1960s I wrote to the chairman of the ethics committee of every county medical society in my state of New Jersey, asking how they felt about patients' use of Master Charge and BankAmericard and the like in doctors' offices. Every one of them wrote back expressing a negative view. Some got a bit emotional, and one carried on for three pages, not only about the lack of ethics exhibited by any physician who would stoop so low as to accept a credit card, but also about my audacity in raising the question.

The responses puzzled me. Those who tried to explain why using the credit card was unethical did so by saying that it's non-professional and commercial. I never did figure out why a plastic card is more commercial than currency or a check.

I do know that the credit card is convenient, often far more so than currency or checks. I find it almost impossible to carry enough currency around with me to get through an average week, much less an average month. The money seems to disappear more quickly than I can get to the bank or friendly neighborhood liquor store, which, being a more pleasant place than a bank in which to transact business and being open for business far more hours each week, may be America's No. 1 financial institution.

Also, my wife, who likes to pay the family bills, prefers a three-to-a-page checkbook. So to me checks are hopelessly inconvenient, because I'm forever forgetting to report back on the use and the amount of the missing checks attributable to me.

That leaves a credit card as a method of payment. I've never lost one. None has every given me any trouble. Traveling without it would be inconvenient; growing numbers of restaurants and other institutions refuse to accept traveler's checks.

For me, the credit card has become a natural and useful part of my financial and personal life. That's true, no doubt, for many other people. Many of us would not be offended in the least by the sight of a bank-card sticker in a doctor's office.

That's not the same as saying that it's ethical for you to display the symbol or accept a card in your office. You must reckon with your county medical society ethics-committee chairman. Yes, the American Medical Association's Judicial Council—it's been called quite erroneously "the Supreme Court of medical ethics"— has approved the use of credit cards for paying doctors' bills, but medical ethics is subject to local determination. In other words, the chairman of your county society's ethics committee is the guy who rules on such matters for you. There's a fair chance that he's not even aware of the Judicial Council's position—or gives a damn about it. So inquire before getting involved with a card plan.

If you do get his green light, you'll find that there are both advantages and disadvantages to accepting credit cards. The chief advantage is obvious enough: You collect right away from many a patient who might otherwise take his own sweet time about sending you a check later. The chief disadvantage is that it costs you money to accept a credit card; the bank or other sponsor usually assesses 3 to 5 per cent of the gross billings charged, the percentage depending on the volume of business handled.

Also, your financial secretary must invest about a minute for each payment by a card. First, she must check the card's expiration date; if she accepts an expired card and the patient fails to pay the bank, you have to absorb the bad debt. She must also check the patient's signature against the signature that appears on the card. Then she must check the card company's bulletin on cancellations and warnings to be sure the card is valid and not stolen.

From a practice management viewpoint, it makes good sense to accept a credit card. The chances of collecting a medical bill or any bill is in inverse ratio to the age of the debt (money owed you for six months is worth only about 67 cents on the dollar), and a credit-card payment is *now.* So, too, is a check or currency and, since accepting either of those costs nothing, your financial secretary should always give them preference when the patient offers a choice. Sometimes, though, the choice is a credit card now or the promise of a check in the mail "later." In that situation, any financial adviser I've ever met would tell you to take the card.

What about jacking up your fee to the patient to cover the fee you pay for letting him use the card? Well, that's exactly what much of the flak is about. Just about everyone agrees that any such action is unethical. This ruling from the Medical Society of the State of New York states the current judicial view succinctly: "A physician may not, because of his participation, increase his fees for medical services rendered the patient."

Somewhat similar in concept to the bank charge-card plan is the cosigned bank loan. This technique has long been in common use among dentists, but only in the mid-1970s did it start finding its way into medical use—largely by big group practices, especially those on the West Coast.

When you cosign a loan, a local bank agrees to pay off the bill of any patient you recommend. After the patient has signed a paper or two, the bank pays you in full, and the patient pays off the bank according to a mutually agreed-on schedule. Banks usually aren't too happy to make such an arrangement for less than $500 or whatever the limit is in its own charge-card plan. They want you to use a credit card for smaller amounts, since the relatively cumbersome bank-loan plan is costly to administer. About 95 per cent

**119**

of cosigned bank loans are paid on time and in full. That's important to know, since you're guaranteeing each loan, and you must return to the bank any defaulted amounts. But that's not really a serious drawback; anyone who'd beat a bank out of its money can be safely presumed to be a patient who wouldn't pay a doctor.

In case you're wondering why I'm beginning this chapter with a discussion of two out-of-the-ordinary ways to deal with patients who are hard to collect from, there's a good reason. It's true that you'll probably collect 95 per cent of your fees—in time. It's also true that the new doctor in town gets far more than his share of deadbeats. Many of your well-established colleagues will be happy to refer their deadbeats to you. And many such patients will find you all by themselves. They must. No other doctor in town will accept them as patients; they've been everywhere else, they've cheated everybody else, and no one else will take them.

Please notice that I'm talking specifically about *deadbeats*— the kind of people who can pay but won't. That kind makes up no more than 1 or 2 per cent of the population, but even that small percentage makes for a long line; there are more than 218 million Americans now. Remember: Deadbeats are people who can afford to pay. They just prefer not to.

That's an entirely different kind of person from the patient you may have thought I was talking about. People who would like to pay but can't because they're poor *are not deadbeats.* They're people who are either temporarily or permanently in situations that make it impossible for them to pay. These patients tend to be very easy to deal with and are usually grateful, so they're welcomed in most practices.

Any patient experiencing some temporary financial bind, as almost everyone does at one time or another, needs time and patience and a reasonable agreement with your office on when and how he's going to pay. Your financial secretary strikes the bargain; you stay out of it, except when there's some special situation that she is unable to handle.

Her attitude, like yours, must be realistic. A professional service has been rendered, and now payment is due on terms that are mutually acceptable. Your fees are based on payment at the time of service by most patients, a minor delay in payment by some, and slow payment by a very few. A patient who promises to pay in a specified number of equal monthly installments starting, say, the second month after he returns to work is a good bet to deliver his promise. Assume honesty. Always. But be sure to put the agreement in writing, so that misunderstandings are avoided.

In some instances, a photocopy of the letter or memo about the agreement—usually signed by your financial secretary rather than by you—can be a useful reminder to pay. Other kinds of collection reminders are widely available from medical cataloguers. Rubber-stamped messages are the cheapest to use and get the poorest results, possibly because they look the cheapest—as if to say you're not serious about collecting. Printed collection stickers often get a better result but not everywhere; they've been used by so many doctors in some communities that they've lost their effect on patients who most often need to be reminded to pay.

Less used and often far more effective are simple printed reminder messages, and these, too, are widely offered by the cataloguers. Bibbero Systems, Inc., for instance, offers an excellent selection for $0.023 a note in pads of 50. Or you can have a local printer prepare a series of customized dunning notes, the wording drawn from the notes that appear in Figure 11-1, which also provides a good schedule for their use.

What about patients who pay their bills routinely? They seldom need reminders. Mostly, they need to know how much to pay. The best time to tell them is while they're still in the office. In many practices, 2 out of 10 patients will pay at the time of service without any prompting whatsoever if they know how much to pay.

Because of that fact, I'm still surprised every time I see a medical office that routinely lets patients out of the office not knowing how much money they owe. This situation is common-place. And I can't imagine a more obvious place to institute better practice management.

The solution is called a charge slip, at least by me. The same little device also goes by various other names—routing slip and patient visit slip, for example. Whatever name it's called by, it's a piece of paper, often with one or more carbonless copies, on which

FIGURE 11-1

# A Billing-Collection System That Works

The schedule outlined below is for routine and ordinary situations, not for special cases. Cases in litigation, cases with special insurance problems, and cases involving patients in temporary or indefinite financial difficulty are among the special situations that require extraordinary handling and good judgment. This schedule is designed for use with patients who can pay but are slow:

| In this month | Example | Send this | And this |
|---|---|---|---|
| When services were rendered | January | Statement | Nothing else |
| Month after | February | Statement | Nothing else |
| Month No. 3 | March | Statement | Note No. 1 |
| Month No. 4 | April | Statement | Note No. 2 |
| Month No. 5 | May | Statement | Note No .3 |
| Month No. 6 | June | Statement | Note No. 4 |

Ten business days after sending Note No. 4, the account can be turned over to a medical collection agency or to an attorney. If the collector fails to collect within six months, consider dismissing the patient from care, using a carefully worded letter signed by you and giving about 30 days' notice.

## Note No. 1

Does your account contain some error? If so, please phone me at once. I'm anxious to keep the account accurate and up to date.

Financial Secretary
(212) 555-1234

## Note No. 2

Please phone me right away. If paying your account in full would be impossible just now, perhaps you and I could work out a satisfactory budget payment plan.

Financial Secretary
(212) 555-1234

## Note No. 3

I'm sure there's some good reason why you've failed to phone me by now or to make payment on your overdue account. Now I must hear from you soon, before the accountants take the matter out of my hands.

Financial Secretary
(212) 555-1234

## Note No. 4

Sorry. Unless you and I can make arrangements for payment within 10 days, your account will be picked up for enforced collection.

Financial Secretary
(212) 555-1234

the patient's name and the services rendered are written.

On completion of the visit, the patient is handed the slip and asked to return it to the financial secretary. She, seeing what services were rendered and knowing the fee for each, strikes a total and says to the patient something like this: "Today's charge is $25. That brings your outstanding balance to $50." In some offices, this sentence is added: "Would you like to pay by cash or by check?" That added sentence is effective, to be sure, but I don't know that it's any more necessary than an expectant expression on the financial secretary's face.

Charge slips are offered by all the medical cataloguers, and they don't cost much. Colwell, for instance, offers them for as little as 2 cents each in lots of 2,000.

More sophisticated versions are a bit more expensive. My favorite is the superbill sold by Bibbero Systems, Inc. It measures 11 by 8½ inches and is printed in three parts—original and two copies. The price—less than 6 cents each when ordered in quantities of 10,000—includes custom imprinting with your name, address, telephone number, specialty, and your selection of standard codes that are widely recognized by insurers as specific definitions for the services rendered.

The point of the superbill is that it doubles as a charge slip and as an attachment to a health-insurance claim form for speedy preparation. The patient's copy can be attached to a claim form for either patient reimbursement or assignment payment to you by the insurer, as you wish. (See Figure 9-2 in Chapter 9.)

The danger of taking the assignment is that you may end up without the difference between your fee and that part paid by the insurer. Your acceptance of the assignment is a signal to many patients that you'll accept the insurance company's check as payment in full, no matter how inadequate the insurer's check is. The alternative problem is that some patients won't pay anything—not even the amount of the check they receive from the insurer.

Most doctors have traditionally gone for the assignment of benefits. In recent years, however, a great many have changed their minds. The trend now is to accept an assignment only on a highly selected basis—or not at all, ever. In some cases, a patient's insurance forms aren't even processed in the medical office until payment for all services rendered has been received. That way, there's no question of accepting an assignment; the patient keeps the insurer's payment, such as it is, as reimbursement to the extent of his coverage.

That way seems a bit tough to me, but I'm not so sure that it isn't justified, especially when it's accompanied by a tactful attempt to re-educate patients. A great deal of health insurance, including Blue Cross and Blue Shield, has been aggressively sold in a way that victimizes doctors. I specifically mean sales pitches that suggest to the patient that the insurance he buys will always cover all his medical expenses.

I wish I could say that that sort of thing belongs to the distant past, but it doesn't; only this month, I saw the same pitch in an insurer's newspaper display ad. Anyone who buys that coverage is going to be damned unhappy when he discovers that his doctor

FIGURE 11-2 ═══════════════════════════════════════════

### The Essence of
### Successful Collections

Collections at the time of service can be almost mechanical when your assistant uses this four-step standard procedure:

☐ **Take pen in hand.** No matter how bold or how shy you are, you need do only that as a mechanical reminder to take this second step:

☐ **Smile.** At the same time, reach for the charge slip the patient is carrying to you. It shows all the services rendered. If the doctor wants the standard fee for each service, he need not enter any figures; he knows you have a list of standard fees in front of you and can enter the figures yourself. While striking the total:

☐ **Speak right up.** "I'll get this statement totaled for you right now, Mrs. Jones," you can say. Getting the total should take only a few seconds. If you have trouble with arithmetic, ask your boss to invest $10 in an electronic calculator.

☐ **Present the fee.** "The charge for today's services comes to $25, Mrs. Jones. Your previous balance was $30, so that brings your balance due to $55." All you need to add now is another expectant smile. In some offices, though, these words are added: "Would you like to pay by cash or by check?"

Remember: A valuable professional service has been rendered, and it's time now that the service be paid for. Nothing wrong with that.

expects a payment from him, over and above the amount paid by the insurer.

In many such instances, the patient has bought an inferior product; it doesn't begin to pay a doctor's full fee. The patient must learn, through the efforts of the financial secretary and the insurance secretary, that the deal is between the insurer and the patient, not between the insurer and the doctor. The patient bought the coverage; his complaint is with the insurer.

If the insurer has misrepresented his product, the insurer should catch the heat; the doctor, not the insurance company, sets the doctor's fees. One way to deliver that message is in person, before the service is rendered. Another way is to deliver it again when the charge slip is presented at the front desk. A third way, if necessary, is in printed payment reminders accompanying overdue bills. As I said earlier, such messages are widely available from the medical cataloguers.

How to prepare your monthly statements? There are a variety of good ways. Possibly the worst is a simple printed statement that says, "For services rendered," followed by the balance due written with a pen or typewriter. If you want payment with minimum fuss, you'd better itemize. A careful listing of every service and its fee is more easily accepted than is a grand total.

An easy and relatively low-cost way to prepare an itemized bill: shingled billing. Like a school tablet, a shingled bill consists of several pieces of paper held together at the top by a gummed edge—three or more monthly statements on carbonless duplicating paper, and attached to a ledger printed on card stock. Both charges and payments can be entered on the outside copy by a typewriter or ball-point pen; they're reproduced automatically all the way through to the ledger copy. The copies are mailed in successive months as the monthly statement. When the bill has been paid in full, the ledger card is filed permanently in the zero-balance file. If the account has not been paid in full by the time the last monthly statement is used, the balance due is entered on a fresh set of shingled bills.

Colwell, New England Business Service, Inc., and Cyril-Scott Company are among the cataloguers that offer shingled bills.

They're available with three, four, or six statements attached to the ledger card.

A much better-known and more widely used way of preparing monthly statements is photocopy billing. Each transaction is recorded on a ledger card—the standard card measures 8 by 5½ inches—and all the cards for patients who need to be billed are photocopied. The photocopies go into the mail. Each ledger card designed for this use has the space for the name and address of the person to be billed in such a position that, when the photocopy is folded, they show through a window envelope. Addressing is thus avoided. So is stamping if you buy your envelopes prestamped. (Bibbero sells them that way. So does the post office.)

Most medical offices that use photocopy billing do their own duplicating. Some, however, buy the service from companies that operate vans with one or two copying machines mounted in the back. The van pulls up to your door on a day agreed to in advance, and the van operator carries your tray of ledger cards to his copier and does all the work there. The good thing about such service is that the work is all done by someone else, and so billing day doesn't disrupt your practice, even though hundreds or even thousands of statements may be prepared in the van.

As a rule, the van operator folds the statements and inserts them into window envelopes, seals and runs the envelopes through a postage machine, and then drops them off at the local post office. All very convenient, simple, quick—and a bit higher priced than shingle billing but lower in price than most other kinds of billing.

The drawback is that the van operator may not do your work when you'd like it done. The best time to put monthly statements into the mail is whenever they get the best results, and you'll get different results in different communities. Almost everyone speaks of getting the bills in the mail by the end of the month or soon after the first of the month. Either time usually produces far better results than waiting until the 5th or the 10th or the 15th. Often, though, the best time is the 20th to the 23rd or the 20th to the 25th. You'll have to experiment to discover what time works best for your practice.

In a variation on photocopy billing, a representative of a billing firm comes to your office toting a portable microfilm camera;

instead of photocopying your ledger cards, he microfilms them. Later that same day, he sends the exposed film to his company's lab, where the film is developed and statements are prepared and mailed. Their appearance is much the same as those produced through photocopy billing.

The advantages are the convenience of having someone else do the work, minimal disruption of your office, and the saving of an investment in billing equipment. The main disadvantage is that it takes a relatively long time for bills to get into the mail. The bigger the gap between the time the ledger cards are filmed and the time the bills are in your patients' hands, the larger the number of payments that will fail to appear on the statements. The omissions mean that angry patients get on the phone or come into your office, demanding to know why your financial secretary failed to give credit for payment.

Despite the cost of the equipment, accounting machines are used in a surprising number of practices. Most accounting machines are mechanical (spring-operated) or electric; some are electronic, often with some memory capacity. These machines work just fine in some practices, but they can be disastrous in others, largely because they require skilled operators.

Whether the machine is a full-fledged computer or something less, at least three trained operators are required—the person who normally operates it, the person who runs it when No. 1 is on vacation, sick, or otherwise absent, and the person who backs up No. 2 when No. 1 is gone. The common error is that no one looks ahead that far or fully appreciates the possibility that No. 2 can get sick while No. 1 is on vacation or that any of the three operators may resign. More often, just one assistant in the office knows how to run the machine, and she always seems to be out sick or threatening to quit because she can be paid much more to run the same machine elsewhere.

By and large, management consultants like me take a dim view of having such a machine in the office. When we see one, we expect to find that entries on ledger cards are routinely posted two weeks or more after the transactions and that monthly statements are routinely in the mail late and with lots of patients' bills skipped.

## Getting started in private practice

Practices farming out the chore to a centralized billing firm that uses either accounting machines or computers get far better results. You'll hear older colleagues curse at the mention of computer billing because of many all-too-true horror stories. For a few years in the late 1960s and early 1970s, just about everyone and his brother thought he could make a fortune by selling computer billing services to physicians. Well, a lot of those firms went down the tube. But the survivors seem to have an excellent record of getting the job done right. That's not to say, though, that you need to avoid a new firm offering the service; sometimes the people who made the old-line firms successful drift away and start their own enterprises.

Also, the minicomputer keeps coming closer each year to making good sense. It's becoming faster, more sophisticated, and ever-lower in price. By the end of the 1970s or soon after, the minicomputer or terminal tied to a larger, centralized computer will probably be snapped up even by one-man practices. The minicomputer will produce your monthly statements, prepare your office payroll, do your bookkeeping and maybe your tax work, replace your appointment book, maybe accept and store all your chart dictation, and probably provide you with month's-end management reports that give you all the information you'll need to make decisions on such matters as expanding your office, bringing in another doctor, hiring another part-time assistant, and buying new lab equipment or an X-ray machine.

Whether you're producing monthly statements for pennies or with the help of a machine priced at $5,000 to $10,000, one fact remains: You'll profit by putting a reply envelope in with each statement. Notice how many bills that you get at your house arrive with an envelope, and notice how much more quickly you're inclined to pay them before you get around to paying the ones with no envelopes. Notice, too, that you're almost always expected to put your own stamp on the return envelope. There's a reason for that: All sorts of double-blind studies have proved that people don't mind putting a stamp on an envelope.

It's very often a good idea, too, to have a special address for the return envelopes—your own post office box or that of your bank. That way, you've got much less worry about someone walking off with a bunch of incoming checks. But use a bank's box only if you find a bank that offers lockbox service. With this service, the bank's employees open the reply envelopes for you, bank the checks for you, prepare a list of payments received, and give you the list, together with any correspondence mailed with the checks. Lockbox service saves time, is often inexpensive, and is almost always well worth seeking out. The trouble with it is simply that it's a difficult service to find; few banks offer it, and fewer advertise it.

Also, it's a good idea to list on your monthly statements a separate phone number that patients can call with any questions about the bill or their insurance. The number can be shared by your financial secretary and your insurance secretary. That way, the calls can be handled with little disruption to your practice, leaving the phone on the appointment desk relatively free of such calls.

And what do you do about hopelessly overdue collections? You could turn them over to a collection agency or to an attorney who's willing to work as a bill collector and then hope that you get favorable results. The collector will probably keep 50 per cent of any bill collected or, alternatively, will charge you a small fee for each account you turn over to him. Either way, don't expect him to collect much, especially if you're doing a good job of billing and follow-up in your office.

Any bill going to a collector is probably six or seven months old, and that's no time to expect a good result. Remember: It's far better to let your staff at the front desk know what services have been performed, so that they can try to collect at the time of service. After that, a conscientious, soundly based collection effort should bring in 85 or 90 or 95 cents on the dollar.

There's no mystery to such a collection ratio; and it's not necessary to get the least bit nasty with anyone, but there is a need to do the job correctly, punctually, and intelligently. That means someone in your office must specialize in billing and collections; and that person must make a continuing study of the subject.

To begin with, she, too, must read this chapter and also Chapter 14, where we'll take up the question of continuing education for medical assistants.

## 12

## Best public relations
## advice you'll ever get:
## Don't be so damned cheap

You *bet* that's a provocative chapter title, and it's there to attract your attention to a big problem you've inherited. After enjoying the highest reputation in his community for generations, the physician now finds that his public image is rapidly being tarnished, and it's up to you to reverse this trend. The onslaught, and I think it's fair to call it that, centers on incompetence, dishonesty, and costs. Witness this front-page article from The New York Times:

> After long considering the incompetent or careless doctor as a rare aberration of minor consequence, the American medical profession is beginning to regard unfit physicians as a serious problem that may account for tens of thousands of needless injuries and deaths each year.
> While most authorities emphasize that the majority of the country's 320,000 doctors are competent and conscientious, they estimate that as many as 16,000 licensed physicians, or 5 per cent of the profession, are unfit to practice medicine. These doctors, they say, should have their li-

censes revoked, be required to undergo further training or practice only under close supervision. . . .

*The New York Times*
Jan. 26, 1976

And these items:

TRENTON (AP)—Atty. Gen. William F. Hyland announced Wednesday that a . . . physician has been sentenced to an 18-month jail term with 14 months suspended for Medicaid fraud.

Hyland said Dr. . . . was sentenced and fined $9,500 by Hudson County Superior Court Judge Frank G. Hahn after the physician was found guilty of 10 counts of Medicaid fraud and one count of obstruction of justice.

Hyland said . . . was only the second doctor to stand trial on Medicaid fraud. Of six other physicians who have been indicted on similar charges, five have subsequently pleaded guilty. . . .

*The Record*
Nov. 26, 1976

WASHINGTON (AP)—Doctors are often accomplices in the distribution of amphetamines and other weight-loss pills to drug abusers, Senate investigators were told yesterday. . . . In 1975, U.S. doctors wrote 25 million prescriptions for . . . amphetamines.

*The Record*
Nov. 12, 1976

WASHINGTON, April 25—A monopoly-like control by physicians of medical services and a frequently "passive" role by patients in purchasing medical care are helping to push health-care costs up at record speed, the President's Council on Wage and Price Stability said today. . . .

The cost increase in the health sector last year was the biggest ever. The Consumer Price Index for services other than health costs rose 7.7 per cent, while the index for health cost went up 10.3 per cent.

This increase, the report noted, now makes health costs 8.3 per cent of the gross national product, and the average American family must spend 10 per cent of its income on these costs.

"To the extent these changes constitute improvements in the quality or delivery of care, price increases

**132**

would not be 'inflationary' in the technical sense," the report said.

"However . . . there is considerable debate whether the overall quality in delivery of the medical care received by the American people has improved in step with the rapid rises in expenditures and prices. . . ."

Rising costs, the report said, cannot be explained by increased labor costs . . . or by increased costs on nonlabor items. In short, it said, the increased cost of doing business—general inflation rates—does not account for health price rises. . . .

The report explored the paradox that in American industry, technology has improved efficiency and lowered manufacturing costs, while in the health sector, technology has improved care and shortened hospital stays but the costs have risen. . . .

*The New York Times*
April 26, 1976

That's the kind of publicity your elders have been getting for years, and increasingly so of late. It's part of their legacy to you, and frankly, there's precious little you can do to control it. Complain to The New York Times or the Associated Press or CBS all you like: Of every 100 readers or viewers who see the attack, maybe 20 will see the retraction or your rebuttal and, of those 20, maybe 5 will be inclined to believe what you say.

To illustrate, let's look at two more excerpts from The New York Times:

ROCHESTER, N.Y.—The public is repeatedly exposed to statistics about medical care. The news is usually bad, rarely encouraging or reassuring. . . .

The New York Times . . . estimated that 938 patients subjected to gallbladder surgery in 1975 were the victims of "avoidable deaths." Is it not strange, then, that the distinguished gastroenterologist editor of The New England Journal of Medicine, on whose pages the statistics first appeared, estimated that the number of avoidable deaths was 113. Estimates that vary by a factor of ten suggest either gross error or puffery. . . .

How can the public guard itself against health statistics that are premature, exaggerated, or patently false? The burden must start with the source of the data, to be both accurate as to his facts and circumspect as to his conclusions and generalizations. But the science writer, too, has an important role to play.

Professional journalistic competence and honesty should involve checking of facts and the soliciting of critical evaluation so that a balanced story results. Finally, the reader must learn to read his newspaper or listen to television coverage with a degree of criticism and skepticism that is proportional to his past experience with being misled by bad reporting.

Louis Lasagna, M.D.
*The New York Times*
May 6, 1976

Eight days later, The Times printed this response from a patient-reader:

To the Editor:

I would like to comment on the . . . article by Louis Lasagna, M.D., . . . in which [he] criticized newspapers for bad reporting of medical statistics. Before the record closes on your five-part medical series, I would like to defend it.

I have been going to doctors a good part of my life, what with children, husband, parents, etc. I can say that, although I have pressured for information, I received none; that, although I have pressured for patient education or communication, I have received none. I have learned that doctors are a secretive group.

Thank goodness The Times did publish those articles. I got *some* information from the newspapers; I got *none* from the doctors. Now I'll make my critical judgments. I *am* skeptical of what I read. At least The Times gave me something to be skeptical about. I can't be skeptical about doctors . . . because as a patient or relative of a patient I am not afforded that privilege.

Yes, the criticism is rough, and it isn't just dreamed up by newspaper writers looking for easy bylines or by a few inevitably disgruntled patients. Doctors' employees, doctors' wives, and doctors themselves are also voicing their complaints publicly.

A nationwide survey of medical assistants conducted not long ago uncovered a good deal of dissatisfaction with wages and fringe benefits paid by doctors. That was no surprise, since the purpose of the survey was to measure employees' satisfaction with their compensation. What was surprising were the complaints volunteered, without prompting, about treatment of patients.

For instance, one medical assistant, instead of indicating her preferences among such factors offered on the questionnaire as good wages, job security, good fringe benefits, and good working conditions, wrote that she felt "sympathy for patients who are mistreated and pushed aside for the rich and wealthy. . . . These are the reasons why I left the medical profession. Doctors should be told to wise up. . . ."

And then there was this example:

> LOS ANGELES—To many women, marrying a physician means financial security and social prestige. To others, however, it means a short, unhappy marriage that ends in divorce. . . .
>
> "Divorce is becoming increasingly common among physicians," said Dr. Edward Stainbrook, a psychiatrist and chairman of the department of human behavior at the University of Southern California medical school. "A generation ago, the divorced doctor was the exception, now he is almost the rule."
>
> . . . While no one, including the Census Bureau and medical societies, has collected statistics pointing toward a high divorce rate among doctors, physicians interviewed agreed that such was the case. . . .
>
> "I got tired of being alone," [a woman recently separated from her doctor-husband] said. "He was always too busy at the hospital to devote any time to me or our son. I had a Mercedes and a house in Bel Air, but I didn't have love and affection."
>
> "Doctors are difficult people to live with because nobody ever says no to them," [said a 44-year-old mother of two who was divorced by her surgeon-husband]. "They are used to having their way at the hospital and they expect their wives to jump to their commands the way patients and nurses do. The problems of a doctor's wife always seem trivial to the doctor."
>
> *The New York Times*
> Oct. 27, 1976

Examples of criticism by doctors themselves abound, but this statement is as damaging as any I've ever had occasion to see:

> A Harvard University report on surgical practices in four parts of the country contends that "far too many" doctors who are not surgical specialists are performing operations while the nation's most qualified surgeons are not busy enough.
>
> The researchers concluded that some doctors who operate, including some surgical specialists, do not perform enough operations to maintain a high level of skill. . . .
>
> The study is part of a scrutiny of surgical practices now under way by professional surgeons' organizations. The self-examination comes at a time when a number of consumer advocates, public health experts, and Congressional committees have alleged that a small but significant proportion of surgery in this country is substandard or unnecessary. . . .
>
> *The New York Times*
> Oct. 21, 1976

As a guy who makes a profession of keeping your career as trouble-free as possible, I'm concerned about the criticism I see in the media. But I'm even more concerned because I know it's consistent with the criticism I hear where you live and practice. On Main Street you'll find there's a lot of dislike waiting to be transferred from your elders to you. Here's just some of what I've been hearing there about doctors:

.From the owner of a store that sells and services photocopying machines:

"No, I don't think I'd say that doctors are good customers. Look around the store. Anyone who knows anything at all about photocopying machines knows we make very little profit per unit and work hard to keep our volume high. A lot of our customers appreciate our approach; many of them do business on the same basis, so they don't have money to throw around. But doctors? My partner won't even talk to them. They're making more money than anybody else in town, but more than anybody else, they bargain for lower prices. And there's no pleasing them. I still do business with them, but lately I've begun to ask myself if it's worth it."

The wife of the owner of a wallpaper and decorating shop:
"Oh, yes, we have lots of doctors here. Actually, we deal

mostly with their wives. I have very mixed feelings about them—especially about the wives, I guess. For the most part, they're very demanding. Nobody else tries to bargain for lower prices. *They* all do. This is a small shop, and we don't make very much money here, so we smile and put up with them as best we can.''

And from the manager of the used-car department of a Cadillac dealership:

"They always identify themselves. They're the only ones who do. I've never once had an executive walk on the lot and say, 'Hi, I'm a big-shot executive; aren't you lucky,' but all the big-shot doctors do it just that way. 'I'm a physician, you know.' Or, 'I'm a doctor, and I can steer a lot of business your way from other doctors.' And they don't know a good deal from a bad one. No matter what the price is, they want the car for less. And no matter how much time you spend with them, they won't buy or, at least, not until they've taken forever to think about it. Well, I've had it with them. I don't even want to talk to them anymore. I'd be just as happy if they took their business elsewhere.''

What to do? The scene you've inherited isn't pretty. If you're going to help clean it up, you'll have to do more than give the highest possible quality of patient care. You'll also have to tend *your* public image when dealing with shopkeepers, employees, and patients. To begin:

1. *Don't be so damned cheap.* You don't have to bargain for everything you buy, and neither does your wife. Neither does the medical assistant who buys supplies for your office.

And you needn't be afraid that everyone you meet is out to gyp you. I think that the biggest reason doctors do get gypped is because of retaliation for their all-too-apparent expectation that they will be.

Your best defense isn't a defensive or antagonistic attitude but rather a little homework done in advance of your shopping excursion. There's no shortage of information on the price of Cadillacs; any well-stocked magazine and paperback book counter offers at least a half-dozen publications that help you get a fix on current going prices of cars, new and used.

For the most part, the prices you see marked on goods

offered for sale on Main Street are the prices people pay. Main Street isn't Mexico or Guatemala or Tangiers; you're not expected to haggle every time you buy something.

And if you pay your assistants as little as you can, you're really kidding yourself. You're sure not acting in your own best interest. We'll discuss that in greater detail in Chapter 13.

2. *Consider: Maybe the critics are right.* It seems to me that anytime there's a public attack on the competence or honesty of doctors, they immediately respond with disbelief—as if there were no bad apples in medicine. Of course there are.

There is, I'm convinced, a strongly growing recognition—at least among medicine's leaders, if not the rank and file—that doctors had better police their own. This news is a welcome major step forward. Proper policing will improve the quality of patient care and, in so doing, will improve your image on Main Street and among patients. The misfits are, as never before, being drummed out of medicine or otherwise disciplined. Medical societies are beginning to demand that their members prove that they're keeping up, and they're reviewing their ethics codes, too.

For instance, the College of American Pathologists, at its meeting in Los Angeles in the fall of 1976, voted to establish a special inquiry committee to investigate charges of professional incompetence or misconduct among its members. The organization's president, Dennis B. Dorsey, M.D., described the committee as "a major step for the college in that it will put us in a sound position in terms of risks."

The pathologists' action helps to point up the fact that the criticism is by no means limited to the rantings of careless newspeople and crazed laymen. Well-reasoned criticism from the medical profession is no farther away than the shelves of your local library. This example from Hospital Practice illustrates the point:

> For years, as medical-care expenditures have risen beyond the rate of inflation, there has been no direct relationship between expense and outcome. Longevity has changed little, and the major illnesses such as malignancy and cardiovascular disease remain unimpeded. Heralded preventive measures such as multiphasic screening and

modification of risk factors for cardiovascular disease yield limited benefit. Illnesses disproportionately affect the poor, major environmental and occupational causes of illnesses receive little attention and less action, and malpractice charges intensify. Clearly, there is a crisis in health care, both in its effect upon health and in its cost.

Simultaneously, medical institutions characterize themselves as excellent. Their personnel and their pursuit of knowledge, they say, represent the epitome of that which is possible. To disturb them by changes intended to alleviate the health-care crisis would undermine their excellence.

This suggests a major contradiction: crisis in the midst of excellence. But there is no contradiction. In the aggregate, medical institutions and practices are not excellent. The self-acclaimed excellence is, in practice, a myth. . . .

In the past 15 years, annual expenditures for health care have almost quintupled. Beneficial outcomes are hard to identify. . . .

Some 30 per cent to 50 per cent of present hospitalization is medically unnecessary. . . . Rising physicians' fees have outstripped those of every other occupation. It is well established that nonphysician health personnel can provide some 90 per cent of primary health care with an effectiveness and patient satisfaction equal to that of the physician, often at less expense. . . . Surgery is excessive. . . .

Professional dominance over the health-care enterprise . . . has perpetuated prevailing practices, deflected criticism, and insulated the profession from alternative views and social relations that would illuminate and improve health care. . . .

Good health science and care . . . demand rigorous analysis and testing of our premises and practices, together with candor between professionals and citizens concerning the results.

A health system that is genuine and efficient rather than ineffective and crisis-ridden requires restructuring of health-care organizations and practices. Then citizens, students, and we will no longer be deceived by uncritical perceptions and false expectations. Then, too, excellence can be more reality than myth, and the exhilaration of accomplishment can return to our work.

Halsted R. Holman, M.D.
April, 1976

3. *Consider what patients think.* There are sure a whole lot more patients' votes to count at the polls on Election Day than doctors' votes, and that's as practical a reason as any to pay attention to what the American people think about physicians. What the opinion polls are showing lately is something plain scary.

A Harris survey in 1966 indicated that 72 per cent of the public placed "a great deal of confidence" in physicians. In a Harris survey conducted in 1976, physicians dropped on the confidence scale by 29 points, more than 40 per cent, and even lost to scientists their traditional top-rated position among professionals.

Medical Economics' patient attitude survey in 1969 found that 86 per cent of the patients agreed that the average doctor "is dedicated to helping people more than anything else." In the 1976 survey, only 52 per cent agreed with that statement.

In a survey reported in 1976 by the University of Utah, doctors were described as too expensive, too wealthy, and too hard to talk with. The loudest complaints in that study were directed at excessive waiting time in doctors' offices—precisely the kind of problem that can be solved through better practice management. The study, like all the studies just cited, points up the importance of taking steps like this one to improve at least your own image in your own community:

4. *Run a good practice.* People don't have to wait. They really don't. In Chapter 18 we'll discuss ways to stay on time. With intelligence, planning, and a workable system, you can handle the routine without making anyone wait. When an emergency arises and knocks your appointment system askew, get word to your receptionist; she can offer patients the alternatives of returning later in the day, being seen another day, or sitting there and waiting. So even then, no one needs to wait for you unless he elects to do so.

Just as busy people today are jealous of their time, so, too, are they informed enough to comprehend the reasons behind your decisions. In your grandfather's day, a physician could say, "Take this medicine, and don't ask questions," and probably get away with it. In your father's day, that kind of doctor could usually get away with such words and the underlying attitude, but he collected a larger undercurrent of resentment than he knew and probably more than he has discerned even yet because, even then, patients were becoming increasingly knowledgeable. Television, which at its best is effective audiovisual education, surely had something to do with that. But so did the publication of increasingly sophisticated books and popular magazine articles on health and doctor-patient relationships.

And don't mistake this increasing level of health knowledge as an invitation to use jargon; increasing numbers of patients are hip to that trick, too. They've seen enough comedians on television to know when an auto mechanic or accountant or doctor relies on his private technical language to snow the customer or to mask the fact that he doesn't know his business well enough to translate into plain English.

5. *Be available.* You probably won't schedule night hours in your office, but where does it say that you can't do so in special situations—for instance, the evening of that day when you had to cancel afternoon hours because of the emergency that kept you at the hospital?

And then there's the phone. We'll discuss it more in Chapter 18, so I need only suggest here that you vow now to accept emergency phone calls just as quickly as you can get to the phone—always—and to return other calls routinely, say, during an unexpected break, or during regularly scheduled call-back periods, both morning and afternoon.

6. *Always wear a white hat.* Never drink when you're on call. And never make passes at patients. If you like to booze it up and chase women, you don't belong in private practice. Get a salaried job; it will give you lots more time off and enough money to live the life you like.

The same goes for dope. There may be more drunks and drug addicts among physicians than in any other occupational group of consequence. I don't say that to be facetious or flip. It's a serious problem.

And don't forget: Good guys never press too hard for collections. Just do the billing-collection routine like clockwork, and you won't have to whip on patients to get them to pay your fees.

Of course, you'll never talk about patients outside the office, because you know gossip spreads like fire. Make sure your spouse knows it, too. One tale told out of class, by either of you, could violate a patient's confidence, put you in breach of ethics, and send your reputation and practice down the chute. It has happened.

7. *Get the best assistants—not the cheapest.* I'll tell you how in Chapter 13; here I want to make sure you know about time-and-a-half for overtime. In the past, almost no doctor paid it, no matter how late he kept his staff. Today, paying time-and-a-half goes beyond public relations and community image. It's a matter of law.

The law holds that you can put management people on salary and work them as many hours as you wish. They may be inclined to quit, but they'll get nowhere trying to sue you for unfair labor practices. However, overworking the rank and file is another matter, and you can't get around it by calling someone "management" when she's not. Plenty of employers have tried that, and they found out that judges aren't stupid.

Don't count on your state's having no law requiring time-and-a-half for overtime work (more than 8 hours a day or 40 hours a week). A Federal law covers such matters, and it applies to any employer engaged in interstate commerce. The definition of "interstate commerce" seems to be expanding all the time. If you see one patient a year from out of state or if you order any supplies or drugs from out of state, you can figure a Federal court will hold you to be engaged in interstate commerce if an employee slaps a lawsuit on you for violation of Federal fair labor standards.

Finally, take time right now and every so often in the future to consider your relationships with your children and spouse. What you've heard so many times before—the kids are small, but you turn around and they're gone—is true. Many an older colleague of yours has never had six serious conversations with his daughter; has never taken his son canoeing or to a ball game or much of anywhere else. And many an older colleague realizes now that he never really knew his wife when she was a young woman.

Increasingly, today's doctor's wife goes back to school after she puts hubby through. She gets her undergraduate degree, and sometimes her master's and maybe her doctorate, all in preparation for a career and an identity of her own. It's about time.

# 13

# How to hire
# the right employees

I wrote a magazine article not long ago on holding down payroll costs, and the editor had a terrible time trying to figure out why I said that the budget for one specialty needs to be different from the budget for another. "Don't you want the same rate of return, regardless of specialty?" he asked.

It's a fair question, and my answer was that budgetary considerations can differ as much from one medical specialty to another as from one kind of business to the next. Just as a supermarket's payroll has no reason to bear any relationship to a travel agency's, there's no reason to suppose that a pediatrics practice must have the same payroll needs as, say, a psychiatrist's office.

In fact, I'm not sure there's any need for the same budgeting even within a specialty. On the average, small-town incorporated general practitioners spend an amount equal to 15.5 per cent of production on office-assistant payroll. But a G.P. with only two examining rooms and little or no lab or X-ray equipment has payroll requirements that bear little similarity to a G.P. in the next town who does all kinds of X-ray and labwork and who sees many geriatric patients in an office with eight examining rooms.

Figures, then, need to be taken with a grain of salt. Nevertheless, it seems useful to know that 15.5 per cent is the payroll outlay for incorporated small-town G.P.s and that incorporated G.P.s in cities with populations of 100,000 or more need to budget 18.1 per cent—a difference of more than 16 per cent. If nothing else, the difference can open a discussion of differences in productivity.

Which brings us to one of the major mistakes made by your older colleagues: They try to make do with too little help. By that, I don't necessarily mean too few bodies. Being on the payroll isn't the same as being useful. I mean too few assistants performing the right tasks.

The key to productivity and to holding down payroll costs at the same time is to practice in a properly laid-out, properly equipped office with the help of the right number of assistants who do the right tasks. And that brings us to the first of nine questions you'll need to answer if you're to hire the right employees?

1. *Specialize or generalize?* In well-managed big group practices—the kind that people generally call clinics—you find people specializing all over the place. In one-doctor practices and even in many with three or four doctors, you find more lone assistants. But an assistant who does everything doesn't do everything; mostly, she does what she wants to do or what she most likes to do. As a result, insurance forms don't get done because they're boring, and monthly statements always go into the mail late.

Well, believe it or not, some people enjoy filling out health-insurance claim forms. Some people in this world think it's fun to do the billing—or any other office task you can think of. Where is it written that you can't find part-time workers who specialize in handling such tasks?

This is precisely where an aggressively managed, member-oriented county medical society can be of use to its members, or you and a few colleagues can join in a cooperative effort. Maybe you can keep an insurance secretary busy a half-day a week but no more. And maybe Joe has exactly the same need, but Harry, who's in a different specialty, can keep her busy four half-days a week. Without looking any further, you know that the three of you have enough work to keep such a woman busy six half-days a week.

Chances are that you can find her—someone who's delighted to pick up three full days' pay a week. She may be too busy with the kids and the house to work any more than that. Or she may figure that you're offering her a good start and that another couple of days' insurance forms will come along in good time.

Specialization is the key to highly productive activity.

2. *Part time or full time?* The key to specialization in a small employment setting like yours is obviously part-time help. But there's an additional benefit: Part-timers get more done per hour of pay than full-timers do.

Fatigue probably has something to do with it. It's easier to go full speed for, say, four hours than for eight hours. You get more production from a morning secretary and an afternoon secretary than from a single all-day-long secretary.

3. *How many assistants?* The number depends not only on how many insurance forms your practice produces in an average week but also on such factors as the number of doctors in your practice, the number of doctor-hours you and your partners spend in the office, and the amount of care given to office records.

Most doctors seem to work best when they work with a specific nurse, rather than with a pool of nurses. Often, there's not much more than make-work for a nurse to do when her doctor is out of the office, so it can make sense to hire someone who's willing to work only when her doctor is in the office.

If that sounds impossible, don't kid yourself; many of your older colleagues work exactly that way. You'd be amazed to discover how many women, including those with some nursing experience, are unavailable for a full-time job but are perfectly happy to work odd hours.

4. *How much to pay?* Everyone, including the housewife who's bored staying home all the time, works for the same basic reason: money. So don't believe anyone who tells you that the money isn't important. It *is*. Given the same set of circumstances

*(Continued on page 152)*

FIGURE 13-1 ════════════════════════════════════════

## How to Hire
## an Assistant

Don't hire lightly. Your assistants can make or break your practice. Selecting them requires thought, underlying data, a plan—a management system. This plan suggests the use of personnel forms from Bibbero Systems, Inc., which provides materials tailored to the medical profession's special needs; at this writing, neither the other medical cataloguers nor the general office suppliers offer materials of comparable scope and quality.

To determine going rates of pay, get in touch with at least two sources—the regional office of the Federal Bureau of Labor Statistics and the administrator of the leading hospital in your area. For going rates of pay for paramedics—physician's assistants, midwives, practicing nurses, physical therapists—try your local or state medical society or state board of medical examiners. One or the other may also give you an idea of the current going rates for new physicians in your specialty. So, too, may your state's specialty society.

|  | Example figures | Your figures | Line |
|---|---|---|---|

**A.** Order basic personnel systems, supplies:
☐ Bibbero catalogue only*
☒ Bibbero personnel systems, forms*    20.50
☐ Wonderlic catalogue only
☐ Wonderlic tests
☐ _____   → **A**

**B.** Nature of job:
☐ Part-time [under 1,000 hours a calendar year]
☐ Full-time [1,000+ hours a calendar year]   **B**

**C.** Title of job:
☐ Business manager      ☐ Group administrator
☐ Office manager        ☐ Appointments secretary
☐ Time manager          ☐ Financial secretary
☐ Insurance secretary   ☐ Chart secretary
☐ General secretary     ☐ General assistant
☐ Physician's assistant ☐ Practicing nurse
☐ Midwife               ☐ X-ray technician
☐ Lab technician        ☐ Nurse
☐ Driver                ☐ Maintenance assistant
☐ _____

☐ First assistant   ☐ Second assistant   **C**

**D.** Describe duties and authority [on separate schedule]   **D**

*See accompanying form

# How to hire the right employees

**Bibbero Systems, Inc.**

36 Second Street • San Francisco, California 94105
Telephone (415) 421-7927

CUSTOM PRINTING INFORMATION
TYPE OR PRINT IN BLOCK LETTERS

**BILL TO:**

Name _____

Address _____

City _____ State ___ Zip _____

**SHIP TO:**

Name _____

Address _____

City _____ State ___ Zip _____

Name _____

Specialty _____

Street Address _____

City _____ State ___ Zip _____

Telephone _____

State License Number _____

Standard Coding for _____
(If special coding is desired, please indicate and attach list)

Where sequential numbering is desired, indicate starting number: _____
(If no number is indicated, we will start with No. 1)

| DESCRIPTION | CATALOG NUMBER | QUANTITY | PRICE | |
|---|---|---|---|---|
| PRICES ARE SUBJECT TO CHANGE | | | | |
| Doctor's hiring manual | MDP111 | 1 | 4 | 75 |
| Applications for position (pad of 25) | MDP110 | 1 | 1 | 95 |
| Interview evaluation (pad of 25) | MDP120 | 1 | 1 | 95 |
| Individual personnel record (pad of 25) | MDP130 | 1 | 1 | 95 |
| Security binder (14 ring) | MDP9000 | 1 | 6 | 95 |
| Employee policy handbook | MDP137 | 1 | 2 | 95 |
| | | | | |
| | | | | |
| | | | | |
| | | | | |
| | | | | |
| | | | | |
| | | | | |
| | | | | |
| | | | | |
| SUBTOTAL | | | 20 | 50 |
| California Residents: Add sales tax. | | | | |
| TOTAL | | | | |

☐ Check enclosed. We ship prepaid.
☐ Bill me later, plus freight.
☐ Please RUSH my order (4 day delivery). Add 15% to custom imprinted items.
Cal., Ore., Wash., Ariz., Ida., and Nev. orders shipped via UPS. All others via parcel post unless otherwise specified.
ALL ORDERS FOR PRE-STAMPED ENVELOPES MUST BE ACCOMPANIED BY CHECK FOR AMOUNT OF POSTAGE

ORDERED BY _____ DATE _____
SIGNATURE

# Getting started in private practice

|  | Example figures | Your figures | Line |
|---|---|---|---|

**E.** Determine going pay rates in area:
- ☐ Nursing and technical: query leading local hospital ☐ ☐
- ☐ Secretarial, other: query Bureau of Labor Statistics regional office* ☐ ☐
- ☐ Physician's assistant, practicing nurse, midwife: query state medical society placement office ☐ ☐
- ☐ _____ ☐ ☐ **E**

*See accompanying form

**F.** Consider these sources of leads to qualified employees:
- ☐ Your present employees
- ☐ Colleagues
- ☐ Your hospital's personnel manager
- ☐ County medical society's placement desk
- ☐ Placement office, local chapter, American Association of Medical Assistants
- ☐ Work incentive program [possible government subsidy; through local office, State Division of Employment Services or Manpower Council]
- ☐ Placement desk, county senior citizens council
- ☐ Local office, State Employment Service [ask about testing services]
- ☐ Employment agencies [see Yellow Pages]
- ☐ Placement offices, nearby assistant training schools, secretarial schools, high schools, community college, other colleges, other technical schools [see schools listed in Yellow Pages]
- ☐ _____
  _____ ☐ ☐ **F**

**G.** Also consider placing a classified ad:
- ☐ Local weekly newspaper
- ☐ Shopping news
- ☐ Daily newspaper
- ☐ County society bulletin
- ☐ Local or state chapter publication of American Association of Medical Assistants
- ☐ _____ ☐ ☐ **G**

|  | Example figures | Your figures | Line |
|---|---|---|---|

**H.** Write your ad, using the following as a model:

MEDICAL ASSISTANT—9:30-1:00, Mon.-Fri., $3.50 hr. Insurance secretary: Do all claim forms, answer patients' queries about coverage, etc. Letter and résumé (no phone calls) to John Q. Doktor, M.D., 123 Main St., Anytown, U.S.A. 07666.

☐ Be specific as to hours, days, pay, job title, duties, how to reply [show your name and address, rather than a blind box number]                                           ☐        ☐        **H**

**I.** Discard misaddressed, sloppily addressed, and sloppily written responses. Of the remainder, select the best three: call or write to them, offering an interview. Also write a "We're keeping your letter on file" letter to all the others.                                           ☐        ☐        **I**

## How to Determine Going Rates of Pay for Clerical Jobs

**J.** Get phone number of the appropriate regional office of the Bureau of Labor Statistics          (212) 971-5405     (___) ___     **J**

**K.** Call: Ask for "median weekly earnings, Table A-1, latest area wage survey" and for "average weekly hours" with specific reference to the following Government job titles [medical-office equivalent terminology is shown in brackets]:

☐ "Secretaries, Class A, Services" [OFFICE MANAGER]; hours:___          $240.00     ___

☐ "Secretaries, Class B, Services" [APPOINTMENTS SECRETARY]; hours:___          $210.00     ___

☐ "Typists, Class B, Services" [PRIVATE SECRETARY]; hours:___          $141.00     ___

☐ "File Clerk, Class C, Services" [CHART SECRETARY]; hours:___          $128.50     ___

☐ "Accounting Clerk, Class B, Services" [FINANCIAL SECRETARY]; hours:___          $156.50     ___

# Getting started in private practice

## Bureau of Labor Statistics Regional Offices

**Region I**
1603 JFK Federal Building
Government Center
Boston, Mass. 02203
Phone: 223-6761 (Area Code 617)

| Connecticut | New Hampshire |
| Maine | Rhode Island |
| Massachusetts | Vermont |

**Region II**
Suite 3400
1615 Broadway
New York, N.Y. 10036
Phone: 971-5405 (Area Code 212)

| New Jersey | Puerto Rico |
| New York | Virgin Islands |

**Region III**
3535 Market Street
P.O. Box 13309
Philadelphia, Pa. 19101
Phone: 595-1154 (Area Code 215)

| Delaware | Pennsylvania |
| District of Columbia | Virginia |
| Maryland | West Virginia |

**Region IV**
Suite 540
1371 Peachtree St., N.E.
Atlanta, Ga. 30309
Phone: 526-5418 (Area Code 404)

| Alabama | Mississippi |
| Florida | North Carolina |
| Georgia | South Carolina |
| Kentucky | Tennessee |

**Region V**
9th Floor, 230 S. Dearborn St.
Chicago, Ill. 60604
Phone: 353-1880 (Area Code 312)

| Illinois | Minnesota |
| Indiana | Ohio |
| Michigan | Wisconsin |

**Region VI**
Second Floor
555 Griffin Square Building
Dallas, Tex. 75202
Phone: 749-3516 (Area Code 214)

| Arkansas | Oklahoma |
| Louisiana | Texas |
| New Mexico | |

**Regions VII and VIII**
Federal Office Building
911 Walnut St., 15th Floor
Kansas City, Mo. 64106
Phone: 374-2481 (Area Code 816)

VII

| Iowa | Missouri |
| Kansas | Nebraska |

VIII

| Colorado | South Dakota |
| Montana | Utah |
| North Dakota | Wyoming |

**Regions IX and X**
450 Golden Gate Ave.
Box 36017
San Francisco, Calif. 94102
Phone: 556-4678 (Area Code 415)

IX

| Arizona | Hawaii |
| California | Nevada |

X

| Alaska | Oregon |
| Idaho | Washington |

## Area Wage Surveys

A list of available bulletins is presented below. A directory of area wage studies including more limited studies conducted at the request of the Employment Standards Administration of the U.S. Department of Labor is available on request. Bulletins may be purchased from any of the BLS regional offices or from the Superintendent of Documents, U.S. Government Printing Office, Washington, D.C. 20402.

| Area | Bulletin number and price* | Area | Bulletin number and price* |
|---|---|---|---|
| Akron, Ohio, Dec. 1975 | 1850-80, $ .45 | Miami, Fla., Oct. 1975 | 1850-76, $ .95 |
| Albany-Schenectady-Troy, N.Y., Sept. 1975[1] | 1850-63, $1.20 | Milwaukee, Wis., Apr. 1976 | 1900-22, $ .85 |
| Anaheim-Santa Ana-Garden Grove, Calif., Oct. 1975[1] | 1850-75, $ .85 | Minneapolis-St. Paul, Minn.-Wis., Jan. 1976 | 1900-3, $ .95 |
| Atlanta, Ga., May 1976 | 1900-30, $ .85 | Nassau-Suffolk, N.Y., June 1976 | 1900-35, $ .85 |
| Austin, Tex., Dec. 1975[1] | 1850-83, $ .75 | Newark, N.J., Jan. 1976 | 1900-10, $ .85 |
| Baltimore, Md., Aug. 1975[1] | 1850-62, $1.30 | New Orleans, La., Jan. 1976 | 1900-2, $ .75 |
| Billings, Mont., July 1976 | 1900-39, $ .55 | New York, N.Y.-N.J., May 1976 | 1900-48, $1.05 |
| Binghamton, N.Y.-Pa., July 1975 | 1850-50, $ .65 | Norfolk-Virginia Beach-Portsmouth, Va.-N.C., May 1976[1] | 1900-27, $ .85 |
| Birmingham, Ala., Mar. 1976[1] | 1900-11, $ .95 | Norfolk-Virginia Beach-Portsmouth and Newport News-Hampton, Va.-N.C., May 1976[1] | 1900-33, $ .85 |
| Boston, Mass., Aug. 1975[1] | 1850-58, $1.50 | | |
| Buffalo, N.Y., Oct. 1975[1] | 1850-69, $ .95 | | |
| Canton, Ohio, May 1976 | 1900-28, $ .55 | Northeast Pennsylvania, Aug. 1976 | 1900-43, $ .65 |
| Chattanooga, Tenn.-Ga., Sept. 1975[1] | 1850-67, $ .85 | Oklahoma City, Okla., Aug. 1976 | 1900-42, $ .55 |
| Chicago, Ill., May 1976 | 1900-32, $1.05 | Omaha, Nebr.-Iowa, Oct. 1975 | 1850-56, $1.10 |
| Cincinnati, Ohio-Ky.-Ind., Mar. 1976 | 1900-7, $ .75 | Paterson-Clifton-Passaic, N.J., June 1976 | 1900-38, $ .55 |
| Cleveland, Ohio, Sept. 1975 | 1850-64, $1.30 | Philadelphia, Pa.-N.J., Nov. 1975 | 1850-65, $ .85 |
| Columbus, Ohio, Oct. 1975[1] | 1850-78, $ .95 | Pittsburgh, Pa., Jan. 1976[1] | 1900-1, $1.15 |
| Corpus Christi, Tex., July 1976 | 1900-41, $ .55 | Portland, Maine, Nov. 1975 | 1850-72, $ .45 |
| Dallas-Fort Worth, Tex., Oct. 1975[1] | 1850-59, $1.50 | Portland, Ore.-Wash., May 1975 | 1850-40, $ .75 |
| Davenport-Rock Island-Moline, Iowa-Ill., Feb. 1976 | 1900-25, $ .55 | Poughkeepsie, N.Y., June 1975[1] | 1850-70, $ .65 |
| Dayton, Ohio, Dec. 1975 | 1850-73, $ .45 | Poughkeepsie-Kingston-Newburgh, N.Y., June 1975[1] | 1850-68, $ .75 |
| Daytona Beach, Fla., Aug. 1976 | 1900-45, $ .45 | | |
| Denver-Boulder, Colo., Dec. 1975 | 1850-82, $ .75 | Providence-Warwick-Pawtucket, R.I.-Mass., June 1976 | 1900-31, $ .75 |
| Detroit, Mich., Mar. 1976[1] | 1900-15, $1.25 | Raleigh-Durham, N.C., Feb. 1976 | 1900-18, $ .55 |
| Fort Lauderdale-Hollywood/West Palm Beach-Boca Raton, Fla., Apr. 1976 | 1900-20, $ .55 | Richmond, Va., June 1976 | 1900-34, $ .65 |
| Fresno, Calif., June 1976 | 1900-29, $ .55 | St. Louis, Mo.-Ill., Mar. 1976[1] | 1900-19, $1.25 |
| Gainesville, Fla., Sept. 1975 | 1850-57, $1.10 | Sacramento, Calif., Dec. 1975 | 1850-87, $ .65 |
| Green Bay, Wis., July 1976 | 1900-37, $ .55 | Saginaw, Mich., Nov. 1975 | 1850-71, $ .55 |
| Greensboro-Winston-Salem-High Point, N.C., Aug. 1976 | 1900-47, $ .65 | Salt Lake City-Ogden, Utah, Nov. 1975[1] | 1850-74, $ .75 |
| Greenville-Spartanburg, S.C., June 1976[1] | 1900-36, $ .85 | San Antonio, Tex., May 1976 | 1900-23, $ .65 |
| Hartford, Conn., Mar. 1976 | 1900-14, $ .55 | San Diego, Calif., Nov. 1975 | 1850-77, $ .45 |
| Houston, Tex., Apr. 1976 | 1900-26, $ .85 | San Francisco-Oakland, Calif., Mar. 1976 | 1900-9, $ .95 |
| Huntsville, Ala., Feb. 1976 | 1900-17, $ .55 | San Jose, Calif., Mar. 1976 | 1900-13, $ .75 |
| Indianapolis, Ind., Oct. 1975[1] | 1850-66, $ .95 | Seattle-Everett, Wash., Jan. 1976 | 1900-6, $ .65 |
| Jackson, Miss., Feb. 1976 | 1900-8, $ .55 | South Bend, Ind., Mar. 1976 | 1900-5, $ .55 |
| Jacksonville, Fla., Dec. 1975 | 1850-81, $ .45 | Stamford, Conn., May 1976[1] | 1900-40, $ .85 |
| Kansas City, Mo.-Kans., Sept. 1975 | 1850-55, $ .80 | Syracuse, N.Y., July 1976 | 1900-44, $ .55 |
| Lexington-Fayette, Ky., Nov. 1975[1] | 1850-84, $ .75 | Toledo, Ohio-Mich., May 1976 | 1900-24, $ .55 |
| Los Angeles-Long Beach, Calif., Oct. 1975[1] | 1850-86, $1.15 | Trenton, N.J., Sept. 1975[1] | 1850-60, $1.20 |
| Louisville, Ky.-Ind., Nov. 1975 | 1850-79, $ .45 | Utica-Rome, N.Y., July 1975[1] | 1850-48, $ .80 |
| Melbourne-Titusville-Cocoa, Fla., Aug. 1975 | 1850-54, $ .65 | Washington, D.C.-Md.-Va., Mar. 1976 | 1900-12, $ .85 |
| Memphis, Tenn.-Ark.-Miss., Nov. 1975 | 1850-85, $ .45 | Westchester County, N.Y., May 1976 | 1900-46, $ .55 |
| | | Wichita, Kans., Apr. 1976 | 1900-21, $ .55 |
| | | Worcester, Mass., Apr. 1976 | 1900-16, $ .55 |
| | | York, Pa., Feb. 1976 | 1900-4, $ .55 |

*Prices are determined by Government Printing Office and are subject to change.

[1]Data on establishment practices and supplementary wage provisions are also presented.

|  | Example figures | Your figures | Line |
|---|---|---|---|
| ☐ "Secretaries, Class D, Services" [INSURANCE SECRETARY]; hours:_____ | $179.50 | _____ | |
| ☐ "Date of wage report?" | 5/76 | _____ | |
| ☐ "Your name and phone extension?" | _____ | | K |
| L. Determine the hourly rate for full-time employment: Divide the weekly wage by the number of working hours | $5.05 | _____ | L |
| M. Determine the hourly rate for part-time, full-responsibility employment: Multiply Line L by 1.07 | $5.40 | _____ | M |
| N. Determine the hourly rate for a first assistant: Multiply Line M by .6 | $3.24 | _____ | N |
| O. Determine the hourly rate for a second assistant: Multiply Line N by .8 | $2.59 | _____ | O |
| P. Be sure your wage rate does not fall below your state's minimum wage: | $2.50 | _____ | P |

## How to Determine Going Rates of Pay for Nursing and Technician Jobs

Q. Ask the personnel manager or the administrator at your hospital to fill in the blanks below. Since he/she may not have the figures immediately at hand, plan ahead; getting them may take two weeks. ☒
Specify: "all day-shift positions" ☒
Also request: "weekly working hours" ☒
Specify: "median or average wages, expressed in hourly rates" ☒ ☐ Q

| | Example figures | Your figures | Line |
|---|---|---|---|
| R. R.N.s; hours; _____ | $6.21 | _____ | R |
| S. L.P.N.s; hours: _____ | $5.00 | _____ | S |
| T. P.N.s; hours: _____ | $5.00 | _____ | T |
| U. X-ray technicians; hours: _____ | $5.24 | _____ | U |
| V. Lab technicians; hours: _____ | $5.05 | _____ | V |
| W._____; hours:_____ | _____ | _____ | W |
| X. Determine employee's hourly rate for part-time work in your office: Multiply hourly rate [$5.05] by 1.07 | $5.40 | _____ | X |
| Y. Determine hourly rate for office-trained nursing assistant: Multiply Line X by .6 | $3.24 | _____ | Y |

but more money in another job, the underpaid worker is long gone.

Your best bet is to pay the median of the going rates in your area. How much is that? Ask your medical management consultant, or get on the phone and chase down some statistics yourself.

To begin, check the phone directory for your state department of labor and industry, dial it, and ask the operator who answers for the prevailing wage unit. If she says there's no such thing, say that you want the going rates of wages for office positions in your community.

You may have to keep explaining to a dozen or so bureaucrats until you're finally connected to the right person. Once you find him, either he'll have the information or he won't. He should; the going rates are determined by recurring statistical research all across the United States; the problem is that some bureaucrats are so unaware that they don't even know the content of reports sitting on their own desks.

If you're lucky, you'll get a marginally knowledgeable state employee on the phone, and you can ask for the going rates for specific job titles. You'll find both the governmental job titles and the equivalent medical-office titles in Figure 13-1, line K, which also shows the going rates in my own community as I write this chapter.

The going rates in your community when you're looking for employees will probably be different. When you know what they are, fill in the blanks in the "Your figures" column. Then get out your pocket calculator and figure the recommended wage for part-time help at Line M. Note that you multiply the hourly rate for full-time employment by 1.07—a 15 per cent increase. Remember that the cost of transportation and work clothing is the same for a part-time job as for full-time employment. Don't fret about the 15 per cent premium; the productivity of part-time workers usually far exceeds that figure, so you'll still make out financially.

A full-time medical-office assistant's job should be advertised at the median figure quoted in the going-rates study. That way, you can take advantage of the training given by some employer whose starting pay was at the low end of the range. It's more costly to run an on-the-job training school than to steal a trained worker. Usually, though, you need not offer the job at more than the median

FIGURE 13-2 ═══════════════════════════════════════════

## Model Letter to Your
## Rejected Job Applicants

A freshly, individually typed letter is best. But if you have a big batch of applications to reject, you may need to prepare a master "Dear Applicant" letter for duplication by bond photocopier or photo offset. Either way, the body of your letter can read something like this:

---

**John Q. Doktor, M.D.**
123 Main Street
Anytown, U.S.A. 07666

For appointment:          Payment inquiries:          If no answer:
(212) 555-1234            (212) 555-1235              (212) 555-1236


July 1, 1978


Mrs. John B. Applicant
321 Main St.
Anytown, U.S.A. 07666

Dear Mrs. Applicant:

I'm grateful to you for taking the time and trouble to apply for the secretarial opening in my office.

Your application was given careful consideration in light of the specific requirements of this job.

I regret to report that another applicant offered experience and training better suited to those requirements.

I will keep your application on file and will call or write to you if a more suitable position becomes available.

                    Sincerely,

                    *John Q. Doktor*

                    John Q. Doktor, M.D.

---

salary. The median figure often yields good applicants, and it's still low enough to allow you to give merit raises later on.

5. *What about fringe benefits?* This is such an important subject that we'll take it up in far greater detail in Chapter 16, but let me say this much here: The more experienced and self-sufficient your prospective employee is, the more likely she is to let fringe benefits be a factor in her decision to join you. Rank beginners seldom have any appreciation of tax-free fringe benefits, partly because they scarcely know anything about them. The beginning of tax sophistication comes with the escalation of one's tax bracket.

Should part-time assistants get fringe benefits? Years ago, the answer to that question by most medical management consultants was a flat No. But things have changed. There are more kids in the job market these days, but they're usually not as good as older workers. Youngsters are scoring lower than ever before on college-aptitude tests and other competence examinations. And fewer of them seem to be work-oriented. So *competent* medical-office assistants aren't always easy to find. The best way to attract them is to offer a better deal than your penny-pinching competition.

So, yes, give both full-timers and part-timers paid holidays and paid vacations. As for other fringe benefits, do what you think you must to get competent help.

6. *Where to find them?* In many communities the best and easiest way to get good assistants is to advertise for them in the

FIGURE 13-3 ══════════════════════════════════════════

### What Well-Established Practitioners Pay Their Help

An established OB/Gyn specialist generally pays assistants an amount equal to 7 to 10 per cent of his production, as do cardiologists, neurologists, orthopedists, psychologists, and thoracic and heart surgeons.

Internists and pediatricians pay 10 to 15 per cent, as do general surgeons, ophthalmologists and urologists.

G.P.s with well-managed practices generally pay 15 to 19 per cent.

(The term "production" means fees or the value of services billed, whether collected or not.)

classified section of your local paper. Often, it's a weekly. Don't let that stop you. Lots of people pay more attention to the small, gossipy weekly than to a daily newspaper.

Line H of Figure 13-1 shows a model ad. Notice that it's very specific as to duties to be performed, hours to be worked, wages to be paid. That way is best. It eliminates most potential applicants who are put off by one or more of those terms without your having to bother with them. Thus, it delivers a higher-quality applicant, at least for your purposes.

Also, notice that the model ad gives the doctor's name and address, not a box number. A growing number of job seekers know that one seldom gets a reply after responding to a blind ad. Many, I wager, are phony—placed by personnel agencies or managers who have no job to offer but who simply want to get an idea of the kind of applicant they can draw under a given set of conditions or at a certain wage offering.

Of course, you can seek your applicants in other ways. The best part about going the newspaper route is that it's impersonal; the people who come up that road to see you assume that many other applicants will be considered. The impersonality makes it easier to say no. But it can't hurt much to ask your county medical society's placement office or executive secretary for any appropriate applications on file. Many societies keep recent applications ready for review by doctor-employers.

One warning: You've got to be careful about encouraging friends or employees to send their buddies to you. That's always a cheap and painless way to get an applicant or two, but it can be hard to say no to your nurse's best friend.

What about using an employment agency? Many doctors have had excellent results with agencies. But the experience depends on the agency. Many seem totally incapable of understanding an employer's needs. Also, many don't fill part-time positions; if that's what you've got to offer, you may be better off relying on that classified ad.

7. *How to screen them?* You'll have to be arbitrary. Don't worry about it.

On several occasions, I've had replies by the dozens to a

single ad, and in each instance I started the screening process by discarding—unopened—every envelope stupidly addressed with misspellings or the like. Also, I throw out all envelopes that are sloppily addressed—smudged, scrawled, whatever. That leaves me

FIGURE 13-4 ═══════════════════════════════════════════════

## One Way to Schedule
## Incentive Compensation for an Assistant

| | | Example figures | Your figures | Line |
|---|---|---|---|---|
| | Employee: _____ | | | |
| **A.** | Target production per year | $100,000 | _____ | A |
| **B.** | Target compensation for assistant per year | $13,200 | _____ | B |
| **C.** | Target compensation for assistant per month | $1,100 | _____ | C |
| **D.** | Bonus factor: Line C divided by Line A | .011 | _____ | D |
| **E.** | Production in last 12 months | $62,123 | _____ | E |
| **F.** | Monthly compensation due this month: Line E multiplied by Line D | $683.35 | _____ | F |
| **G.** | Salary paid this month | $400.00 | _____ | G |
| **H.** | Balance of compensation fund available for bonus or other fringes: Line F less Line G | $283.35 | _____ | H |
| **I.** | Balance brought forward from Line L, last month's report | $345.67 | _____ | I |
| **J.** | Total compensation fund now available: Add Lines H and I | $629.02 | _____ | J |
| **K.** | Additional compensation elected now by employee: | | | |
| | Bonus _____ | | | |
| | Retirement _____ | | | |
| | Health plan _____ | | | |
| | Group life insurance _____ | | | |
| | Other: _____ | | | |
| | Total | $600.00 | _____ | K |
| **L.** | Balance forward to Line I, next month's report: Line J less Line K | $29.02 | _____ | L |

with envelopes addressed by applicants who cared enough to be neat and accurate. That's the minimum attribute required, I figure.

After opening those envelopes, I compare the letters, again discarding some on sight. Of course, I keep in mind the job that's offered. If I'm looking for a maid or a janitor, I don't need an English major or a secretarial-school graduate, but I do look for signs of competence and care.

Then I put all the discarded applications in one pile, and the live ones in another. All the discards receive a stock letter as soon as possible; a model rejection letter is shown in Figure 13-2. The live applicants are asked, by mail or by phone, to come in, fill out an application, and be interviewed.

8. *How to hire them?* Here's where the Bibbero forms come in handy—the ones we discussed back in Chapter 9.

To begin, there's the hiring manual, which gives complete details on how to conduct the interview and all the rest. One of the three basic forms in the Bibbero package includes a form that takes you step by step through both the interview and the subsequent reference investigation. Another form is the job-application blank, which is created specifically for use in the medical office. It's terrific, and it's designed to meet the standards of the Fair Employment Practices Act.

I'm also impressed by some of the testing materials offered by E. F. Wonderlic & Associates, Inc.; they're especially good for practices with more than one or two doctors. For about $30 Wonderlic can provide enough tests to screen the number-perception and typing skills of 25 applicants. The tests are described in Wonderlic's free catalogue, which is available on request to the company's home office at 820 Frontage Rd., Northfield, Ill. 60093.

And that brings us to this final question to consider:

9. *What risks to watch out for?* Don't take the Federal anti-discrimination laws lightly. Doctors have already been hit with lawsuits because of them. And the Federal laws may be the least of your worries, tough as they are. Many states are now actively policing job discrimination, and many state laws are tougher than the Federal laws.

There are all sorts of Federal laws. Title VII of the 1964 Civil

Rights Act, as amended by the 1972 Equal Employment Opportunity Act, is the basic law from which all the subsequent legislation has sprung; it covers employers of 15 or more persons, including part-timers. It prohibits discrimination because of race, color, religion, sex, or national origin in any term, condition, or privilege of employment. Employers with 25 or more workers must also worry about the 1967 Age Discrimination in Employment Act, which outlaws job bias against any applicant in the 40-to-65 age bracket.

But don't think you're off the hook because you employ fewer than 25 or 15 people. Title VI of the 1964 Civil Rights Act prohibits job discrimination based on "race, color, or national origin in all programs or activities that receive Federal aid." That includes Medicaid and Medicare.

The various state laws match the Federal laws or go much further in establishing the definition of fair practices. The best way to find out about your state's current job-discrimination laws is to phone or write to your state department of labor in the state capital or at the regional or local office. There's a good chance that you'll find it's against the state law to discriminate on the basis of physical or mental handicaps, weight, or, of course, sex.

But don't be put off by all that. There's one sure way to avoid any problems in your hiring and employment practices, and that's to recruit, pay, promote, and fire your employees because of only one factor: ability to perform the job. To prepare, you'll need to decide exactly what a new employee's duties are to be. Write them down. Use the list routinely when screening your applicants. And think twice before asking an applicant any personal questions that have nothing to do with job performance—especially questions concerned with such matters as handicaps, medical condition, race, religion, national origin, marital status, pregnancy, having or not having children, sexual orientation, and gender.

# 14

# How to get intelligent work from your employees

I used to roam the country doing practice surveys and other one-shot assignments, such as setting up partnerships and corporations. Now I provide monthly continuing services to clients, and I don't get a chance to see nearly as many doctors and doctors' offices as I used to. Nor do I see the surprising. That's the part I kind of miss.

For instance, there was the time I opened a closet door in a corridor off the X-ray room in a Pennsylvania office and stepped back as, Fibber McGee-style, patients' films by the thousands came tumbling out. The X-ray technician in this busy orthopedic practice hadn't filed a piece of film since her assistant resigned, nearly two years earlier (it was the assistant's job to do the filing). Instead, the technician had tossed each new addition to the top of the precariously balanced stacks inside and quickly closed the door.

Similarly, in a big practice in Louisiana, I started opening overhead cabinets in what was called the accounting room and discovered more than a thousand patients' ledger cards with charge slips clipped and stapled to them. None of these charges had been posted, and none of those patients had been billed—for periods ranging up to a year. The lone assistant assigned to do such work couldn't begin to keep up with it, and I also learned that she was afraid to ask the doctor to hire more help.

And then there was the three-doctor practice in Oregon that hadn't billed a single patient in four months. Nor had an insurance form been prepared in that time. In that practice, every office assistant was supposed to drop her regular duties once a month—on billing day—and get those monthly statements in the mail. And, in theory, everyone chipped in to prepare the insurance forms. The problem was, of course, that everyone's job was no one's job.

You may as well face it: Many people hate filing, bookkeeping, or any once-in-a-while work that gets in the way of the work they like. On the other hand, it's almost impossible to name a task that someone doesn't love. Remember "Honeymooner" Ed Norton? He worked in the sewer because he wanted to.

None of those classic blunders nor any of the scads of others I've seen would have occurred if the doctor-employers had appreciated the need to make a business of being a boss. If you don't boss intelligently, don't expect your staff to perform intelligently. Supervision is a career all by itself, so you'll have to know at least some of the basics. To begin, digest these six points:

1. *Determine in advance exactly what work an assistant is supposed to do.* As your practice grows, it's not enough simply to hire one person for the front office and one for the back.

I can't begin to give you all the potential job titles that you'll find in your office years from now, when your modest enterprise has grown to a staff of 118 full-time positions and an auxiliary staff of opticians, traveling nurse-practitioners, midwives, physician's assistants who staff satellite and mobile offices, computer analysts and programmers, among others. But long before you reach that point, you'll have an appointments secretary (to book your patients and schedule your time); a financial secretary (to tally the charge slips, ask patients for money, and keep your financial records); a charts secretary (to transcribe your dictation and prepare reports and letters to other doctors); a private secretary (to keep your traveling schedule straight, prepare your correspondence, and type your speeches and articles); and an insurance secretary (to prepare all your health-insurance claims forms and give talks all over the state to medical assistants eager to learn how to do such work better and more quickly). And, of course, each of those secretaries will have assistants to help cope with the growing workload, and an office manager will supervise their efforts, hire and train and evaluate them, and fill in whenever any one of them is absent.

Unless you're fiercely determined to remain in solo practice for the rest of your career, you'd do well to assume that you'll eventually have assistants in at least four of those basic job categories—appointments, finances, charts, and insurance. A private secretary and an office manager may be needed in time, but help in the other four areas is needed the day you enter practice. And that's just in the front. I haven't even gotten around to talking about a nurse, an X-ray technician, a lab technician, or whatever your particular practice will require in the back.

At the start, you may decide to have one assistant do everything, front and back. But that decision depends pretty much on your specialty. If you do most of your work at the hospital, if you have no lab or X-ray facilities in your office, and if the nursing function amounts to little more than escorting an occasional patient from the reception room to the consultation or examining room, you can probably get by with only one assistant.

But if you're in a specialty that requires a great deal of activity and patient care in the office—family practice, internal medicine, pediatrics, OB/Gyn, orthopedics, ophthalmology, allergy, or preventive medicine—you'll find your staff expanding just as rapidly as your practice. So be clear about the duties each one is hired to perform.

2. *Hire enough assistants, and try to see that each has sufficient capability to get the job done.* There was a time when almost no employer would willingly hire someone overqualified for a job. It was assumed that smart people do poorly in undemanding jobs.

Then came the economic uncertainties of the 1970s, and some employers began to see that growing numbers of smart, well-educated folks were going hungry because there was a lot more easy but tedious work than challenging work available. So they hired smart people for low-level jobs.

Well, neither way makes any sense. You can't generalize much when hiring. You've got to use your best judgment on an individual basis, and you've got to try to find the best person among your limited pool of applicants to fit the specific job. If it's important—and it is—to figure out just what the duties are before you even advertise the position, it's equally important to make every reasonable effort to see that the person who appears to be most capable of handling the assignment is the person you hire.

The selection process is more a test of your intelligence than that of the applicants. You needn't fret, though, about turning people away. Saying no isn't pleasant, but wouldn't you hate to say yes to someone not qualified for the position?

For many years, all too many people who do the hiring have tried to find mechanical substitutes for good human judgment. Some mechanical substitutes do make sense—typing tests and the like. If a person is being hired to do nothing but type, it makes sense for her to demonstrate some ability to type. On the other hand, you don't need to use intelligence, aptitude, and personality tests; some are only good for keeping lots of personnel specialists and industrial psychologists busy and employed.

Intelligence alone never gets the job done. Performance is a combination of ingredients that can never be usefully measured, because they change, even from day to day, with all the internal and external pressures that can alter one's motivation and capabilities—working conditions, tools for the job, and good or bad supervision included.

So you'll never be able to read or hear or see or study enough on the subject to fully understand personnel administration. But you can quickly adopt some guidelines.

For instance, you'll probably discover early in the game that you love your work and take great delight in working with people who enjoy your company, are pleasant, and have the same sense of professionalism that you do. Once you've defined your own attitude, you'll have a chance of recognizing it in others—job applicants, for instance.

3. *Establish priorities for your assistants and for the office.* The first priority is to bring in the money. You're involved in a money-based economic system, and you're in a business that won't be around long and thus won't long be of any service to anyone if it doesn't bring in the money. That's basic.

You'd think that point would be obvious to everyone, but it isn't. The most common problem I've seen among office managers is almost total disregard for such mundane chores as determining fees, keeping financial records, billing, collecting, and preparing insurance forms.

Is it their fault? Right. But it's the doctor-employer's fault, too. He obviously failed to establish priorities.

4. *Provide opportunities for continuing education.* Among medical assistants, there's a general lack of emphasis on the kind of professionalism that leads to a continuous upgrading of job skills.

Every good doctor I've ever met or heard of makes a lifelong study of his profession. I strongly suspect, in fact, that there's a direct relationship between a doctor's income and the amount of time he puts into continuing education, sharpening his ability to diagnose and treat. And yet this doctor seldom encourages the same kind of professional interest among his staff members.

There are five basic ways for assistants to keep up. First, they can go back to school for courses directly related to present or future assignments in the office. To encourage this, pay at least half the course fee, on condition that it be taken for credit and that the final grade is A or B.

Second, there are seminars. In the mid-1970s the American Medical Association started to give seminars and workshops for medical assistants in various parts of the country, often in co-sponsorship with a state or county medical society. Medical management consulting firms are becoming more and more involved in management workshops for medical assistants. Also, a number of other medical or doctor-related organizations—Medical-Dental Hospital Bureaus of America, to name one—sponsor programs. And several nonmedical organizations, such as the American Management Association, put on programs of potential value. You'll find lots of programs announced in your so-called junk mail.

**Getting started in private practice**

A third way to upgrade skills is to join a continuing-education organization. Perhaps the best one available for medical-office assistants of all kinds is the American Association of Medical Assistants. Its purpose is continuing education, and it's interested in both the clinical and the business sides of medical practice.

A fourth way: self-study. This way is getting easier all the time. Medical Economics Book Division offers "Your Roles as a Medical Assistant" and "Aid for the Medical Assistant," each at $8.50, and is preparing to publish a series of handbooks for medical assistants in winter 1978. The Institute for Management provides all sorts of materials that can upgrade supervisory skills; its "I.F.M. Workshop for Supervisors" costs $19.95. Schrello Associates offers financial audiocassette courses; "Collecting Money by Telephone" costs $69.95. General Cassette Corporation recently came out with a two-cassette course for appointment secretaries, "Effective Telephone Techniques for Secretaries and Receptionists," which costs $35; it also offers college-level review courses on such subjects as business management, child development, mental hygiene, and social psychology for as little as $2 each. And Learning Dynamics sells such audiotape educational courses as a 12-program series on human behavior, covering such topics as how to handle difficult people and how to solve problems; the course sells for $119.70, about $10 a program.

What I like about such materials is that they can become part of an ongoing educational library of value to both present and future assistants. Also, they can be introduced at and made a part of the monthly staff meeting, which is the fifth basic way to encourage continuing education in the office. To be effective and to keep from degenerating into gripe sessions, the monthly staff meetings must be strongly directed toward the goal of improving office procedures and individual skills. Each assistant can report briefly every month on new developments she has become aware of in her area of specialty.

For instance, the insurance secretary should go through Medical Economics magazine for any new tips on processing health-insurance claims forms. She, like every other assistant, should maintain a file or a three-ring binder of magazine articles

**164**

addressed to her specialty, plus notes and reports on information and techniques learned at seminars, workshops, American Association of Medical Assistants meetings, whatever.

5. *Get rid of bad apples.* Believe me, a staff of professionally minded assistants who are interested in their work and in improving their skills and the efficiency of the office want people with the same motivation added when you do more hiring. An assistant who can't or won't cut the mustard needs to be replaced before her presence adversely affects office morale.

But be very careful whenever you let someone go. You could be asking for a lawsuit if you do anything wrong.

For example, all the legal considerations discussed in the last chapter with regard to hiring also apply when firing. In other words, you can't fire on the grounds of race, color, religion, age, national origin, or gender. To do so is to ask for lots of bad publicity and a very big fine because of Federal and state employment-practices legislation.

Also, you ask for a lawsuit for defamation, libel, or slander if you write or say anything derogatory that you can't prove in a court of law. You'd better not fire someone because you think she's embezzling if the district attorney doesn't first agree that you've got enough evidence to convict her. If you don't have that evidence, you probably don't have enough evidence to beat any lawsuit she brings against you for telling someone—and it need be only *one*—that you fired her for stealing.

Remember that warning, too, when a potential employer phones or writes you and asks about her. You're under no legal obligation to tell him anything, much less anything that could get you into trouble. If you can't speak well of her, don't speak at all. If you're pressed to explain why she left, you're probably on safe ground if you say that she was a good worker whose skills would be far more useful in an office larger (or smaller) than yours or that the problem was nothing more important than a personality conflict, which probably wouldn't be repeated in a different setting with a different combination of people, or that times are tough, you had to lay off somebody, and she drew the short straw.

Mind you, I'm not telling you to lie. I am saying that you dare not speak derogatorily unless what you say can be proved in court. With a little creative thinking, you can come up with a fair though mild (and nonactionable) explanation.

How much termination pay should you give a fired employee? Well, she's already earned some pay in lieu of paid vacation days accrued. You've got to pay that much. In addition, some severance pay is only fair, it seems to me, since you had the bad judgment to hire her, rather than some better choice. I suggest one week's pay (with appropriate payroll deductions) for each year of performance, with a minimum of one week for anyone who's been on your payroll as long as three months. In the case of part-timers whose pay tends to fluctuate from one week to another, calculate the average weekly pay for the last three months or so.

Oh, you don't like to fire anyone? Very few employers do. Just remember: Out there somewhere, looking for work, is someone who needs the job, wants the job, and can handle it like a pro. Why deprive *her*?

6. *Give them sound guidelines.* It's up to you to set policy, and you've got to set it if you want to be in control—and you have to be. You're in the business of earning your living as a physician in private practice. Not one of your employees is in the same business as you. Each one of them is in the business of earning a living by being a nurse or a secretary or whatever. It's natural that she do it the easiest possible way—unless you make it clear that a higher level of competence is expected and will be rewarded and that you'll tolerate nothing less. In that light, an employee's efforts to fulfill her own needs are far more likely to fulfill yours as well.

After the frequent restating of directions, priorities, and responsibilities, what's left comes down mostly to ongoing supervision—the kind that not only bosses your employees but also keeps them satisfied and working for you. And that's exactly what we'll discuss in the next chapter.

# 15

## How you're gonna keep 'em (happy) down on the farm

The most financially successful doctor I've ever met had the single biggest problem I've ever seen: his office manager. She was just like most office managers. She wanted to do a good job, but she didn't have the foggiest notion how.

The doctor is so well known in his specialty that I'm reluctant to reveal it or even his part of the country. No matter. His problem evolved exactly the same way it does in smaller practices. In that sense, his problem is classic.

His office manager had progressed the natural way. She had been his first employee when he got out of training and opened shop. For a while, she worked both the front and back office, and even at the start there were many days that she had to spend at full gallop. She came to the medical field with no prior experience in it, but she learned quickly enough to do what she had to do to get by—fetching and carrying, preparing patients for examinations, answering the phone, greeting patients, and, when they were fin-

FIGURE 15-1 ═══════════════════════════════════════

## Model Letter Requesting Help
## From an Assistant Who Resigned

Many medical offices suffer all sorts of ills wholly unknown to the doctors there—supervisory or other personnel problems that make employees unhappy, create costly turnover in staffing, and impede practice growth. When an employee leaves a big company, he's likely to be asked to sit down with an executive for an exit interview—a confidential discussion of why he or she is leaving. The executive may be the employee's supervisor's boss or someone completely separated from his department—someone in the personnel department, for instance. Big companies can't afford the disruption caused by a rapid turnover of employees; therefore, many of them make this special effort to identify as early as possible a situation or person who may be at fault so that the problem can be corrected.

You can't afford such disruption, either. You may need to conduct your own exit interviews. If you don't have the chance, you can send the departed employee a letter something like this one.

---

**John Q. Doktor, M.D.**
123 Main Street
Anytown, U.S.A. 07666

For appointment:          Payment inquiries:          If no answer:
(212) 555-1234            (212) 555-1235              (212) 555-1236

Aug. 1, 1978

Mrs. Susan Hughes
543 Main St.
Anytown, U.S.A. 07666

Dear Susan:

I do wish we'd had a chance to discuss your resignation in private before your departure.

I'm concerned that your resignation may have been prompted by some condition here in the office that made it unattractive to stay any longer—some fault of mine, perhaps, or of others.

This should be a happy place in which to work. If it is not, I need your help to make it so.

I'd be most happy to hear your suggestions.

Sincerely,

*John Q. Doktor*

John Q. Doktor, M.D.

---

ished, showing them out the door. Right from the start, she was reluctant to stop the daily routine even once a month to put the bills in the mail, and somehow talking on the phone had always kept her from completing an insurance form.

As the practice grew, the need for additional help became obvious. His assistant had a say in the hiring of the second woman in the practice and each one after that. Typically, she, being the first woman in the social unit, viewed the doctor as a kind of Dad and herself as a kind of Mom, and so the second and all subsequent employees were her kids. Her rule was absolute. Anyone who failed to treat her deferentially or who was equally aggressive or was anywhere near as smart soon found herself without a job.

Mom, unfortunately, had the brains of a loaf of pumpernickel. The little family she gathered around her was not to be believed. Every one of them was pleasant, but it's hard to find anything else nice to say about them. The doctor was such an incredible diagnostician that the blunderings and fumblings of his pleasant dunderheads couldn't hold him down—at least, not that you could notice. His production was more than seven times the national average.

But collections were something else. I was astonished when I saw how much money was being lost because of missed billings and a host of other reasons.

"That woman has been pleasant to you all the years you've been in practice," I said, with the idea of talking him into getting rid of her, "but in all that time she's failed to improve her job skills. While you've become one of the two most respected physicians in your specialty in this country, her inability to handle the billing, collecting, and insurance forms is losing you the equivalent of one Cadillac every two and a half weeks." I put it that way because I'd already learned that the man is a Cadillac freak.

Well, I got his attention and then a look of disbelief. I trotted out the figures and proved my point. I hadn't been exaggerating. He shook his head sadly and said his office manager would have to go. I told him how to make a deal with one of the local hospital administrators to have her installed in a job there.

"If necessary," I suggested, "offer to reimburse him for part of her salary. In fact, reimburse him for all of it, if you must. You'll be money ahead even then, just by keeping her out of your office."

Well, looking back, I think now that I should have appealed to his social conscience. I could have figured out how much he might have lowered his fees by collecting 95 per cent instead of 65 per cent of his production, and by rebuilding his staff with equally pleasant but competent, productive workers. I suspect the savings to patients would have been considerable.

## FIGURE 15-2

### A Sampling of Producers

Since it's easy to spend $100 or more for an audiovisual training program, you need to shop carefully and look into the possibility of cooperative purchasing. A training library is a good idea for tenants in a medical arts building or in offices along doctors' row. It's also a good idea for a county medical society or a state or professional society. Some of the places to check for applicable audiovisual training materials are these:

#### AUDIO CASSETTE

☐ P   Educational Design, 47 West 13th St., New York, N.Y. 10011
☐ N   Career Aids, 229 North Central Ave., Glendale, Calif. 91203
☐ P   AuViCation, 1150 West Olive Ave., Burbank, Calif. 91506
☐ C   Western Tape, 2273 Old Middlefield Way, Mountain View, Calif. 94040
☐ N   Robert J. Brady Co., Bowie, Md. 20715
☐ CP   BNA Communications Inc., 5615 Fishers Lane, Rockville, Md. 20715
☐ G   Management Resources Inc., 757 Third Ave., New York, N.Y. 10017
☐ M   Automated Learning Inc., 1275 Bloomfield Ave., Fairfield, N.J. 07006
☐ M   Learning Systems Co., 1818 Ridge Rd., Homewood, Ill. 60530
☐ G   American Management Association, 135 West 50th St., New York, N.Y. 10020
☐ G   Nation's Business, Executive Seminars Div., 1615 H St. N.W., Washington, D.C. 20062
☐ C   Lanier Business Products, 1700 Chantilly Dr. N.E., Atlanta, Ga. 30324
☐ SO   Medical Economics Cassette Service, Oradell, N.J. 07649
☐ G   E.F. Wonderlic & Associates, Inc., Box 7, Northfield, Ill. 60093
☐ —  
☐ —  

I can hardly begin to say how many things were wrong in that practice because of the office manager. The saddest part is that this particular situation wasn't much different from many others I've surveyed. The numbers were just bigger. The doctor, mind you, was a giant in his field—internationally respected and for good reason. Had he been merely average, I wondered, would he have remained in private practice? Under those office personnel condi-

---

## of Training Materials

### FILMSTRIP

| | | |
|---|---|---|
| ☐ | NO | Audiscan, Box 1456, Bellevue, Wash. 98009 |
| ☐ | N | AuViCation (address under Audio Cassette) |
| ☐ | N | American Sterilizer Division, Erie, Pa. 16512 |
| ☐ | GP | Better Selling Bureau, 1150 West Olive Ave., Burbank, Calif. 91506 |
| ☐ | N | Robert J. Brady Co. (address under Audio Cassette) |
| ☐ | N | Edmark Corp., 655 South Orcas, Seattle, Wash. 98108 |
| ☐ | PN | Harris-Tuckman, 751 North Highland Ave., Hollywood, Calif. 90038 |
| ☐ | N | Setco Audio-Visual, 4400 St. Vincent Ave., St. Louis, Mo. 63119 |
| ☐ | N | Train-Aide Educational Systems, 1015 Grandview Ave., Glendale, Calif. 91201 |
| ☐ | NO | Trainex Corp., Box 116, Garden Grove, Calif. 92642 |
| ☐ | T | Zapel Studios Co., 615 North Wabash Ave., Chicago, Ill. 60611 |
| ☐ | — | |
| ☐ | — | |

### PRINTED MATERIALS

| | | |
|---|---|---|
| ☐ | M | Medical Economics Book Division Inc., Oradell, N.J. 07649 |
| ☐ | SO | Practising Law Institute, 810 Seventh Ave., New York, N.Y. 10019 |
| ☐ | GP | Behavioral Sciences Newsletter, 60 Glen Ave., Glen Rock, N.J. 07452 |
| ☐ | M | Dow Jones & Irwin, 1818 Ridge Rd., Homewood, Ill. 60430 |
| ☐ | — | |
| ☐ | — | |

KEY: **C:** clerical and business office **N:** nursing and technical **P:** interpersonal relationships, handling people **L:** clinical **S:** personal finances, investments, taxes **T:** telephone handling **O:** other **G:** supervision, management **M:** comprehensive

---

FIGURE 15-3 ═══════════════════════════════════

## Job Description

Each employee can write her own job description and update it from time to time, perhaps on the same day each year. Keep it on file—the original in a filing folder; along with all the other job descriptions, so that you can review them when it's time to add to your staff or replace someone. A copy can go in a ring binder maintained by the office manager or another assistant. The binaer should contain a section for each job, and each section should contain the job description, checklists, and instructions on handling key assignments.

---

Job description

JOB TITLE: Chart secretary No. 1
Section: Business office
Supervisor: Office manager
Date of original description: 9/15/76     By: Jane Flynn
Date of last revision: 9/15/77     By: Jackie Smith

1. Transcribes from cassette transcriber using shorthand or speedwriting or typewritten notes.
2. Prepares final-draft documents from transcribed material.
3. Maintains correspondence files.
4. Supervises No. 2 file clerk in absence of No. 1 file clerk.
5. Supervises No. 2 chart secretary.
6. Supervises No. 3 chart secretary.
7. Reviews work of Nos. 2, 3 chart secretaries; provides job-performance evaluation on either, on request of office manager or doctor-administrator.
8. Maintains list of office temporaries trained to fill in for chart secretaries 1, 2, or 3; provides office manager with an up-to-date listing.
9. Receives, opens first-class mail; sorts, distributes it.
10. Counts checks and money orders received daily; reports total to office manager; turns them over for processing to No. 1 financial secretary.
11. Arranges all doctors' travel schedules; makes reservations for travel, lodging, local tours, meetings, seminars.
12. Prepares all doctors' manuscripts, from transcription to delivery of final draft; maintains manuscript files.
13. Fills in for office manager in her absence.
14. Performs special assignments given from time to time by office manager or, in her absence, by doctor-administrator.

---

tions, possibly not. But he surely would have been motivated to become the kind of supervisor that I'd like to see you be. I hope that you will adopt the following recommendations.

1. *Go slow in choosing an office manager.* An office manager spends all her time hiring, firing, training, and supervising the other assistants, both front and back. That's the theory. More often, the job comes to something less than that, but that's the way things ought to be, according to most management consultants. I don't especially agree. It seems to me that management systems aren't nearly as important as the abilities of the people involved. A really good team can make just about any system work.

So it doesn't bother me in the least if an office manager heads up the front-office staff, and all the assistants in the back answer to a head nurse. If the office manager and the head nurse can make things work, why not?

Nor does it bother me in the least if, in a small medical office, the office manager doubles in brass as the chief appointments secretary or as the financial, chart, insurance, or private secretary. A lot of work needs to be done before a small medical office can afford to have someone on the payroll doing nothing but hiring, firing, training, and supervising. For that reason, it doesn't bother me to see no office manager at all.

In a small medical office, there's no reason why the doctor or doctors should relinquish the hiring and firing task. With the help of those personnel practices and policies discussed in the last chapter, training becomes a group function that requires light supervision. And if each assistant truly takes a professional interest in her assignment, overall staff supervision becomes a small matter, too.

What's left is finding people to fill in for someone who's out sick or on vacation, and the best solution to that problem isn't an office manager, anyway. What you need is either a staff of part-timers or a pool of regular office temporaries. The great feature about a staff of part-timers is that there's almost always one person who can fill in for an absentee by working an extra half-day or two. The standby office temporaries work the same way as substitute teachers; when one is needed, she's called in.

And when an assistant is going to be out sick, she doesn't

## FIGURE 15-4

## Employee Evaluation

Small, frequent raises are a good policy for employees who've been with you less than two years. A quarterly performance review is a good idea for them—the main purpose being to determine the suitability of compensation and assignment. After two years, a semiannual or annual review is acceptable. Be sure to enter review dates on your desk calendar and to review when scheduled. Doctor-employers tend to forget and to lose valued employees through inattention. One system calls for an evaluation and recommendation by the employee's immediate supervisor and the office manager, business manager, or management consultant, plus an evaluation and decision by the doctor-administrator.

Employee: *JACKIE SMITH*
Position: *CHART SECRETARY No. 1*
Review date: *9-15-78*
Period covered: *SINCE 9-15-77*

Reviewers of job performance:
A: *JANE FLYNN, OFFICE MANAGER*
B: *MARGE CORCORAN, MGMT. CONSULTANT*
C: *DR. DOKTOR*

**EMPLOYEE JOB-PERFORMANCE EVALUATION CHECKLIST**

☑ Job description accompanies

**CONFIDENTIAL**

ENTER a 5 for excellent, 4 for very good, 3 for adequate, 2 for questionable, 1 for poor, 0 for very poor. Enter your evaluation figure in your own column, A, B, or C.

| | A | B | C | COMMENT |
|---|---|---|---|---|
| JOB KNOWLEDGE | 3 | 3 | 4 | |
| QUALITY OF WORK | 3 | 2 | 2 | |
| QUANTITY OF WORK | 4 | 3 | 4 | |
| INTELLIGENCE | 3 | 3 | 2 | |
| ADAPTABILITY | 5 | 5 | 4 | |
| SELF-SUFFICIENCY | 4 | 3 | 4 | |
| VERSATILITY | 2 | 2 | 2 | |
| INITIATIVE | 5 | 5 | 4 | |
| ATTENDANCE, PUNCTUALITY | 5 | 5 | 5 | |
| COOPERATION | 5 | 5 | 5 | |
| DISPOSITION | 5 | 5 | 5 | |
| DEPENDABILITY | 5 | 5 | 5 | |
| DEDICATION | 5 | 5 | 5 | |
| MANAGERIAL POTENTIAL | 2 | 0 | 1 | |
| Totals down | 56 | 51 | 52 | |
| Grand total this review | 159 | | | |
| Grand total last review | 141 | | | |

ADDITIONAL COMMENT:
JF: Fine in present assignment. Recommend small merit raise.
MC: Agree
JD: Ok — 5% increase starting 10-1-78.

have to call an office manager. There doesn't even need to be one person assigned to take such calls. A buddy system can work just as well. Just have the sick one call her assigned buddy or, if she's sick, too, call a standby.

The buddy approach can help get you past the Momism—the dreadful family-like kind of organization—that has bogged down many medical offices. But if you don't need a Mom running things for you out there, neither do you need a sergeant major. If some women make the mistake of organizing everything under the sun as an echo of the family unit, far too many men organize everything to resemble a military unit. In private medical practice, forget it. Your better alternative:

2. *Run it like a team.* Think of yourself as the player-coach. You're a pro; your assistants are all pros. You specialize in what you do; each of them specializes in what she does. Increasing your own skills through continuing education is a big thing with you, and it's also a big thing with each of them.

That kind of a team can do very well for itself. It doesn't need a chain of command.

3. *Be a good boss.* Go to the monthly staff meetings as a participant. Remember: You're the player-coach. Make your monthly progress report, too.

Your assistants don't need to know how to do what you learned to do at that last medical seminar you attended, but they should know you attended it and, in general terms, what you got out of it—and how the new knowledge may affect the way certain patients are now to be prepared for examination and how they may be benefited.

Your monthly report at the staff meeting can be a source of professional inspiration to others on your team and, on occasion, may elicit a suggestion—a tip on a new course or a book of potential value to you, for instance, passed on to you as a result of something said at the last American Association of Medical Assistants chapter meeting.

Also, if your employees are expected to act like pros, then treat them like pros. Treat each one like the expert and specialist she is or will become.

**175**

Listen attentively; that's a sign of respect.

Back up your workers. Never criticize one in front of another, much less in front of a patient.

Watch your temper. Cool gains respect. Hot does not.

Live up to your promises.

Never play favorites.

Always be on the watch for good, new books and workshops on personnel supervision. Until you've read at least one of those books and have been to at least two workshops, you'll never know how good a boss you are.

4. *Run a good staff meeting.* Keep it short and sweet. Don't let anyone get the idea that your monthly meeting is a social gathering. It doesn't have to be held over breakfast or lunch, though it can be. It can just as easily be held in the office as out.

Plan your own participation. You're always studying, so you'll always have something to report.

Demonstrate. Use audiovisual aids when they're appropriate. Pass out photocopies, booklets, whatever.

Report. Don't teach.

Give ample advance notice of the time and place, and start your meeting on time. If anyone's late, never let it be you. If you're held up by some emergency, get the word back to the office as quickly as you can. You don't want employees wasting your time, so don't waste theirs.

5. *Pay for what you get.* So far, we've discussed keeping your staff happy and in your employ by doing what it takes to keep them as professionally involved in their careers as you are in yours. In truth, I think that's the most important part. But not for one moment do I downgrade the importance of paying for proficiency.

Down through the years, your colleagues have shown little appreciation for the need to acquire, develop, and keep first-rate assistants. But your professional life is going to be much better than theirs. You'll inspire and instruct, you'll lead and admire, you'll provide paid time off equal to the standards of your community, you'll pay at least as well as the median employer there, your productivity and that of your office will very likely be the highest in town, you'll probably get through your working day with less expenditure of energy, you'll be surrounded by people who'll make your own working day a joy, and your career will be satisfying.

Since medical-assistant pay and fringe benefits are important to you, let's take a full chapter to discuss them next.

Oh, my doctor-client, the one who's letting all those Cadillacs slip away—well, he still has that office manager. I talked with her on the phone just the other day. I swear, I think I'm starting to like her more. Later, I spoke to her boss and asked him why she's still working there.

"I didn't have the heart to let her go," he said. "Besides," he added, "it's all my fault, not hers. She never asked to be put in charge. She became top dog because—well—I just let things bump along. It was all pretty mindless, and now I've got to pay for being a bad administrator. I guess I was lost in the clinical side of my practice and didn't pay much attention to the other side."

Well, O.K. Seems like an odd way to punish oneself, but he'll get no more nagging from me. I've helped him think his problem through, and I've given him the choices. The decision's his. And he's not at all the bad manager he thinks he is. He's mastered one of the basic rules of practice management: Be the best you can be in your specialty. He sure is. And he always wears a white hat, too.

# 16

## Tax-deductible fringe benefits for your assistants—and for you

I should have known better, but it took a problem in a client's office to awaken me fully to the need to tell employees about the value of their fringe benefits.

The problem's name was Joyce, and she was as good a medical receptionist and office manager as I've seen. She worked for a busy two-doctor practice. Every morning she handled the reception desk and telephone. In the afternoon, she tended to her managerial duties and assigned either of two other women to the front desk.

Largely because of my urgings, Joyce not only joined the American Association of Medical Assistants (A.A.M.A.), but also started working diligently in preparation for the grueling tests required by the organization to become a Certified Medical Assistant (C.M.A.). Across the United States, there are only about 5,000 C.M.A.s, fewer than one per county.

Joyce was one of about eight members of the local A.A.M.A.

**179**

chapter preparing for the next C.M.A. test, which is administered twice each year—regionally, on the first Friday each June; nationally, in the city where the national organization holds its annual meeting in September or October (the date varies from year to year). One of Joyce's friends in the chapter happened to mention to her boss, an orthopedist, that the two of them were going to Chicago for the 1976 convention and hoped to pass the test there.

The orthopedist was fascinated. He hadn't paid much attention to the A.A.M.A. activity in his own office, though two of his assistants were members. He quickly learned that the organization's sole purpose is continuing education. It's been in existence since the 1950s, and annual study-meetings are held not only by the national organization but also by 46 state chapters (all except Delaware, Idaho, North Dakota, and Wyoming), supplemented in some areas of the country by regional meetings. In addition, many local chapters hold monthly meetings, also for purposes of continuing medical education, both clinical and business-office.

Well, we know how demanding orthopedists can be. This fellow wanted to know why everyone in his office wasn't a member of the A.A.M.A.—a question that possibly had something to do with the fact that all his other assistants became members at the next monthly meeting. He also said that hiring in the office would henceforth be limited, when at all possible, to members of the local chapter—even if that meant stealing a key medical assistant from another doctor.

And so, two months later, when his office manager's husband was transferred to the West Coast, Joyce was offered the job of office manager in the orthopedist's busy office—for a 25 per cent salary increase, from $11,700 to $14,625. That would have put Joyce on top of the salary totem pole in her part of Florida.

Well, my client was upset. He didn't like the prospect of losing Joyce, especially to a man he instinctively disliked. But he was also upset with me. The $11,700 salary he was paying was a lot more than he'd once wanted to pay, and he had raised Joyce's salary only on my insistence that he do a better job of protecting himself against the departure of his key people. Now he was mad because I hadn't set the new salary high enough.

But he hadn't yet seen the full extent of his problems. Not 10 days after phoning me the first time, he phoned back to say that Joyce now had an even better offer, this one from a patient of his, of all people. My client, it seems, had complained to this fellow about a colleague's efforts to lure the still-undecided Joyce away with promises of greater riches. The patient, an entrepreneurial type who owned some commercial real estate in the area and an electronics assembly plant out on the edge of town, seemed fascinated, asked questions, got all the answers, and ended up so impressed with Joyce's managerial abilities and interest in improving her job skills that he raised the bidding to an even $15,000. Joyce swooned. My doctor-client very nearly dropped dead.

I didn't like seeing my client so upset, but I really wasn't too unhappy about the situation. I quickly devised a checklist, which I mailed to Joyce and, on its arrival, discussed with her by phone. It's a worksheet that certainly proves that salary isn't the whole story— not by a long shot. The fringe benefits can count for plenty.

Fortunately for my client, the orthopedist had scarcely heard of fringe benefits. He didn't believe, for instance, in paying people for time not worked, and Joyce would have gotten only three paid holidays and one week's vacation. Surprisingly, the entrepreneurial executive's terms weren't much better. The upshot: Joyce decided that she couldn't possibly afford to work for either man.

Her ego-building experience is useful because it shows that fringe benefits are good not merely for the employees but also for the doctor-employer. Liberal benefits can help keep a good staff together, help keep good assistants in the medical field, and quite conceivably lead to gains in office productivity by keeping morale and job interest high.

That's not to say you should jump for any kind of fringe benefit that comes fluttering through your door. I take a dim view of some. I think a well-rounded program of benefits should do the following:

1. *Encourage your staff's efforts to improve.* Joyce was tickled to death to discover the A.A.M.A. Her employer hadn't known of it till I mentioned it, and she hadn't known enough other medical-office employees to learn of it independently. The word from

**181**

FIGURE 16-1 ══════════════════════════════════════════

## Job Budget

You can budget any job—even one with an incentive bonus tied to practice production. Just target your production and the compensation for the job, then project the amount of incentive bonus likely to be drawn in the year ahead. Use a worksheet something like this one.

| | Employee: | Example figures | Your figures | Line |
|---|---|---|---|---|
| A. | Target production per year | $165,000 | _____ | A |
| B. | Target compensation for assistant per year | $13,200 | _____ | B |
| C. | Target compensation for assistant per month | $1,100 | _____ | C |
| D. | Bonus factor: Line C divided by Line A | .00667 | _____ | D |
| E. | Production in last 12 months | $162,457 | _____ | E |
| F. | Monthly compensation due this month: Line E multiplied by Line D | $1,083.59 | _____ | F |
| G. | Salary paid this month | $400.00 | _____ | G |
| H. | Balance of compensation fund available for bonus or other fringes: Line F less Line G | $683.59 | _____ | H |
| I. | Balance brought forward from Line L, last month's report | $345.67 | _____ | I |
| J. | Total compensation fund now available: Add Lines H and I | $1,029.26 | _____ | J |
| K. | Additional compensation elected now by employee: Bonus _____ Retirement _____ Health plan _____ Group life insurance _____ Other: _____ Total | $600.00 | _____ | K |
| L. | Balance forward to Line I, next month's report: Line J less Line K | $429.26 | _____ | L |

her boss prompted her to make a phone call to the county medical society, which knew all about the local chapter.

But my client, whom I'll call Dr. Neff, did everything to encourage a staff continuing-education program and got Joyce to organize monthly staff meetings on paid time, along the lines we discussed in Chapter 15. And, of course, he attended the meetings himself, saw that each assistant was assigned to review one of the socioeconomic magazines coming into the office, and provided not only a meeting time but a place as well—his consultation room, since there was no employee lounge or meeting room in the old office. (He's since moved into a new and bigger place, and it has a meeting room.)

2. *Contribute toward your staff's continuing education.* Chuck Walsh—a medical management consultant in Elmhurst, Ill., a suburb just west of Chicago, and a past president of the Society of Medical-Dental Management Consultants—once told me that he thinks an alert, well-managed practice should budget an amount equal to about 7 per cent of employees' payroll for their continuing education. In later conversations with my management colleagues, I've found that there's no consensus on the figure, but no one seriously quarrels with Walsh's 7 per cent rule. The main point emphasized by my colleagues is that the amount, whatever it is, needs to be budgeted.

Dr. Neff does, indeed, budget 7 per cent of his medical-assistant payroll for continuing education. It's spent mainly on reimbursing his employees' A.A.M.A. convention expenses. But he also earmarks some of the money for books and other teaching aids, including filmstrip programs, which we'll discuss in some detail in Chapter 19.

"You're right," Dr. Neff told me after his conversion to belief in liberal personnel tactics. "A dollar spent toward continuing education for my medical assistants is just as important as a dollar spent for my own continuing education. Why should I be the only one in this office who works hard at getting better?"

3. *Give them plenty of paid time off.* I advised Dr. Neff, just as I'm advising you, to let your A.A.M.A. people go to their conventions on company time, when required. Actually, that's not such a

big burden. Local meetings are usually held in the evenings after office hours and sometimes even on Saturday afternoons and Sundays. State, regional, and national meetings are often built around weekends.

As for paid holidays, you can afford to be liberal, if you can close your office for them. Which ones? Well, for sure, New Year's Day, Memorial Day, Independence Day, Labor Day, Thanksgiving, and Christmas.

Taking off the Friday or Monday before or after any of those holidays is largely a matter of local option, but the tendency now is to create three-day and four-day weekends on almost any pretext.

Lincoln's and Washington's Birthdays are iffy, especially where the employer is liberal in granting those long holiday weekends. Christmas Eve and New Year's Eve depend mostly on the specialty; many practices are so quiet after noon on those days that doctors and employees alike wonder why they hadn't had the foresight to announce half-day holidays in advance.

Employers are taking care of the religious-holiday question by adding two paid personal days off to the paid-holiday list, letting each employee decide whether to take off Ash Wednesday, Passover, Good Friday, Rosh Hashanah, Yom Kippur, or Hanukkah.

As for paid vacations, I start with the premise that no employee is expected to work more than five days a week unless she's paid by the hour or works for time-and-a-half for any portion of the sixth day and for any hour above 40 in one week. Also, I think it should be standard policy to advise prospective employees of the vacation policy before they decide whether or not to accept employment in your office.

That way, there's little disappointment if the policy specifies no paid vacation days in the first calendar year of employment if one goes on the payroll on June 1 or later. If an assistant starts work earlier, grant five days of paid vacation during that first calendar year. In year 2, 10 days of paid vacation are usually competitive—and the same for years 3, 4, and 5. In the sixth to the ninth years, 15 days are justifiable, as are 20 days in the tenth year and thereafter.

Regional differences need to be taken into consideration, of course, and so you need to be aware of your own local competitive pressures. You probably needn't pay much attention to the fringe benefits offered by small employers, including doctors. Your real competition comes from business and industry. So first find out who the best employers in your community are, and then find out what kind of fringe benefits they offer. If you don't number any of their employees among your patients, don't be shy about picking up the phone and calling the personnel director of each company. Chances are that your forthright explanation of your need for the information will be met with cooperation.

If not, you can always call the local office of your state's Department of Labor and Industry. Ask the switchboard operator for the prevailing wage unit. If the operator expresses bewilderment, your state probably uses different terminology. In that situation, just say, "I'd like the going rates of wages for office positions in our area." The bureaucrat who knows the going rates should also be up on the going fringe benefits—at least, those benefits related to paid time off.

4. *Pay some of their health expenses.* Here's where I get a little less liberal. I've heard many medical assistants complain (in private, of course) that free health care had been presented to them as a condition of employment but that they seldom got any. "Are you kidding?" they say. "He's always too busy to look after his own wife and kids, let alone us!"

I believe in discounting services, but I don't believe in giving them away free. Professional courtesy got so out of control in many areas that it's now a thing of the past in some specialties. It's tough, for instance, for psychiatrists to treat doctors and their families without charge; not many of these no-fee patients are needed to fill a significant portion of the day's appointment schedule. The same sort of problem can befall the pediatrician, ophthalmologist, or almost any other practitioner who has the misfortune to keep an office in the section of town where all the doctors live.

The rapidly developing policy almost everywhere is for each doctor to carry full health insurance and for the treating doctor to accept whatever the insurance pays as payment in full.

*(Continued on page 188)*

FIGURE 16-2 ═══════════════════════════

## How Much Is the Job Really Worth?

| | Example figures | Your figures | Line |
|---|---|---|---|
| Employee: _____ | | | |

**A.** List the value of your fringe benefits:

| | | | | |
|---|---|---|---|---|
| Group term life insurance premium | $ _____ | | | |
| Disability insurance premium | _____ | | | |
| Health-insurance premium | _____ | | | |
| Health-expense reimbursement | _____ | | | |
| Any other personal insurance premiums | _____ | | | |
| Convention or study-expense reimbursement | _____ | | | |
| Educational benefit trust | _____ | | | |
| Uniform allowance | _____ | | | |
| Retirement-plan contribution (employer) | _____ | | | |
| Other: _____ | _____ | | | |
| Other: _____ | _____ | | | |
| Other: _____ | _____ | | | |
| Total: | | $ 5,000 | _____ | A |

**B.** Your tax bracket · .25 · _____ · B

**C.** Tax factor: Line B multiplied by 2 · .50 · _____ · C

**D.** Tax savings to you: Line C multiplied by Line A · $ 2,500 · _____ · D

**E.** Total value of fringes: Add Lines A and D · $ 7,500 · _____ · E□

**F.** In addition, these benefits not included above:

| | | | |
|---|---|---|---|
| Number days paid holidays yearly | _____ | | |
| Number days paid vacation yearly | _____ | | |
| Number days sick leave yearly | _____ | | |
| Other paid time off: _____ | _____ | | |
| Other paid time off: _____ | _____ | | |
| Other paid time off: _____ | _____ | | |
| Total: | | 25 | _____ F |

**G.** In addition, the employer pays these expenses, which would be tax-deductible by you in any event but would nonetheless reduce your available personal income:

## Consider Fringes and Taxes, Too

| | | Example figures | Your figures | Line |
|---|---|---|---|---|
| Malpractice insurance premium | | ____ | | |
| Professional car expenses | | ____ | | |
| Professional travel/entertainment expenses not listed at Line A | | ____ | | |
| Other: _____ | | ____ | | |
| Other: _____ | | ____ | | |
| | Total: | $ 7,050 | ____ | G |

**H.** Also, though of no immediate direct benefit to you, your employer pays these taxes because of your employment:

| | | | | |
|---|---|---|---|---|
| Social Security tax | | ____ | | |
| Federal unemployment tax | | ____ | | |
| State payroll taxes | | ____ | | |
| Other: _____ | | ____ | | |
| | Total: | $ 1,148 | ____ | H |

**I.** Gross pay before payroll deductions:

| | | | | |
|---|---|---|---|---|
| Salary or wages | | ____ | | |
| Overtime pay | | ____ | | |
| Bonus: _____ | | ____ | | |
| Bonus: _____ | | ____ | | |
| Bonus: _____ | | ____ | | |
| Other: _____ | | ____ | | |
| | Total: | $25,000 | ____ | I |

### Summaries

**J.** Total of employer's outlay directly to you for pay and fringes other than paid time off: Add Lines A and I — $30,000 ____ J

**K.** Your compensation package, including reimbursement of expenses: Add Lines G and J — $37,050 ____ K

**L.** Clear cash value to you of that package, including taxes you save through the fringes: Add Lines D and K — $39,550 ____ L

**M.** Budget by employer for your job, including employer's share of payroll taxes; excluding funds to replace you during vacations or other absences: Add Lines H and L — $40,698 ____ M

## Getting started in private practice

For hospital and medical-office employees, the tendency is to accept whatever the insurance company will pay or to give totally free care. The better alternative is to accept the insurance.

*Group* health insurance is often the common benefit offered to medical-office employees, and it's almost always unappreciated. Some employees are covered by the family protection provided by their husbands' employers. When that's the case, you're just paying for needless, duplicated coverage. The solution is to provide cash reimbursement of health expenses.

For example, Joyce's plan in Dr. Neff's office was reimbursement to a maximum of 3 per cent of her salary—$351 a year. To collect, she had to pay a physician's or dentist's bill, show Dr. Neff that it had been paid in full, and collect that amount—up to $351 in one year—from Dr. Neff.

The insurance package in the employee-benefit plan was spelled out in Dr. Neff's professional corporation's minutes, but it needn't have been. The I.R.S. has probably never opposed an employee-benefit plan established to reward only the garden-variety employees. It's the plan that benefits the boss that the I.R.S. really gets fussy about. In Dr. Neff's plan, each employee chose whether she wanted an amount equal to 3 per cent of her salary used to reimburse her for major-medical insurance, excess-limits major-medical insurance, hospitalization, medical-surgical protection, hospital-money coverage, dental insurance, disability insurance, or any special insurance coverage, such as the one covering cancer expenses.

His plan, please notice, included reimbursement of disability insurance premiums; most professional corporations separate that coverage from health-cost reimbursement. Notice, too, that health-reimbursement plans can include not only the cost of insurance protection but also the direct cost of care by a physician or dentist— in short, any goods or services normally qualifying as tax-deductible in the eyes of the I.R.S.

What about an employee-benefit plan that covers members of the employee's family? If natural children are to be included, what about foster children? And what about parents or grandparents of the employee and her husband? Well, that's one of the major advantages of the health-expense reimbursement plan: It can easily accommodate any or all or none of those persons, as the employee elects. Expenses are reimbursable, in any event, only to the stated limit—in Joyce's case, $351 for a calendar year.

5. *Pay for life insurance.* Let's get this straight right now: There are two kinds of group life insurance, and a lot of insurance salesmen know only about the first kind. That's known in the trade as true-group, and it covers 10 lives or more. The premium is established by the insurance company's actuarial department. I don't much care for that plan, because I've yet to see the true-group plan that provides as much protection or costs as little as the *de facto* plan I propose.

This second kind of group plan isn't devised by some insurance company; it's a group plan because it's called that in the notice posted on the bulletin board in the employees' lounge, in the personnel-policy handbook that every business office should keep in plain sight, and in the professional corporation's book of minutes. Since all this is a basic part of professional-corporation administration, we'll get into a fuller discussion in the next chapter. Here, though, is the essence:

An incorporated group may purchase its coverage from two different insurance companies—yearly renewable term insurance in amounts of $50,000 or more on each doctor-employee and five-year renewable term protection for each garden-variety employee in an amount not less than 10 per cent of any doctor's coverage. The reason for the two kinds of coverage is simple. Yearly renewable term insurance is often unavailable for amounts less than $50,000, but five-year renewable *is* available in the smaller amounts—though not necessarily from the same company.

6. *Go easy on the paternalism.* A doctor in an office neighboring that of a client of mine in southern California once made a big deal of the fact that he hauled his employees and their families on vacation with him each year. Once he took everyone to Hawaii, all on his nickel, of course. Another time they all went skiing in Colorado. The local paper made a big thing of the doctor and his plan, and I suppose that made him happy. But the medical assistants and their families weren't so pleased.

Not that they hadn't liked the idea at the start. It sounded like a fun trip—all one big, happy family and all that. The trouble was that these women had to work with each other 50 weeks a year, and it took a couple of trips to show them that they didn't need to be in each other's hair for the two vacation weeks. In fact, three of the five women in that office resigned after the skiing trip.

Their reasons probably only partly concerned the need to get away now and then from the people one sees every day. Paternalism is costly, and there's much less of it in American capitalism today than, say, a century ago because employees always figure out that the money spent by Big Daddy might well have been put to better use—like cash in the pay envelope. People work because they need the money, not because they're looking to join a lodge.

7. *Provide a retirement plan.* You don't have to be a professional corporation to provide a retirement plan for employees. The point of a corporation, as we'll discuss in the next chapter, is that it permits the boss to gain *employee* fringe benefits. But if you choose not to incorporate, you can set up an employee retirement plan with an individual retirement account (I.R.A.) or a Keogh plan.

Any employee who isn't covered by an I.R.S.-approved retirement plan can open an I.R.A. Almost everyone knows that an employee can set up such a plan at almost any bank in town, and tax-deduct his contributions to that plan. But not many people also know that the boss can set up an I.R.A. plan for all or any of his employees at his discretion. And he can make all or any part of the contributions to each plan. His contributions are tax-deductible as business expenses and must be shown on each employee's W-2 statement as salary.

Thus, your contribution is additional income to the employee, but she can tax-deduct the whole amount as a retirement-plan contribution. The plan costs her nothing in taxes; it just complicates her income-tax return.

Beware, though: An employer-contributed I.R.A. is a special kind. Make sure your banker knows that such a plan exists. If his bank doesn't offer it, try another bank.

Also, remember that I.R.A. plans are offered by mutual funds and other financial institutions. Perhaps one of them can convince you that the I.R.A. plans in your office ought to be handled by them. However, you can probably get 8 per cent compounded at no risk by signing up with a commercial bank, savings bank, or savings and loan association.

And just in case you're asked, $1,500 invested annually at 8 per cent interest grows in five years to $8,000, in 10 years to $21,729, in 15 years to $40,728, in 20 years to $68,641, in 25 years to $109,657, and in 30 years to $169,920. The funds can be withdrawn either in a lump sum or in monthly increments beginning at age 59½; the withdrawals must begin by age 70½. With increment withdrawals, the interest continues to build up tax-free.

Let's not forget that point, since it's more significant from a tax standpoint than the tax-deductibility of the contributions. All the money saved or invested in such a plan compounds totally free of income taxes. With compounding, interest earns more interest—all tax-free until withdrawal.

And, of course, as the amount invested each year rises, so does the amount of interest earned. That brings us to Keogh.

That's what everyone calls this retirement plan. It's pronounced KEY-oh, and it's named for Eugene Keogh, a Congressman from Brooklyn who offered the enabling legislation many times before getting his bill passed by Congress in 1962. The law has been liberalized since then and will probably be liberalized again under the seemingly never-ending pressure of inflation.

Today, Keogh continues to be the name of the tax-deductible retirement plan available to an employee-owner. Only in Keogh legislation is there any such animal; elsewhere, you're either an employee or an owner or each at different times or in different situations but never both at the same instant, as here. The Keogh legislation invented the employee-owner for its own purposes.

Traditionally, an owner could gain employee status and, therefore, employee fringe benefits only when he was an employee of a corporation, including a corporation he owned. Mr. Keogh's law altered the basic concept, much to the dismay of the I.R.S., by creating the employee-owner status for sole proprietors and partners, thereby giving them some special retirement-plan benefits.

The first of these benefits is the tax-deductibility, today, of

**191**

$7,500 or 15 per cent of earned income, whichever is less. For a self-employed doctor earning $50,000 a year or more from his practice, that means an annual tax-free contribution of $7,500, which can grow at 8 per cent in 25 years to $548,287. To an $11,700-a-year employee like Joyce, it means an annual tax-free contribution of $1,755, which can grow at the same rate of interest over the same period of time to $128,299.

As in an I.R.A., money in a Keogh retirement fund may be taken out, in whole or in part, starting at age 59½; withdrawals must begin no later than age 70½.

If you think that's a dandy retirement plan, you're right. Keogh is good for doctors, and it's good for medical assistants, as is the I.R.A., since many employees, even in the late 1970s, still have no retirement plan at all.

And that's exactly why Joyce stayed with Dr. Neff. The orthopedic surgeon who had offered her a higher-paying job wasn't incorporated, and he didn't have a Keogh plan or even an I.R.A. plan for himself, let alone for his employees. The entrepreneurial executive who had offered her an even higher-paying job did have a corporate retirement plan, but Joyce could never have qualified for it. Under its terms, she, like any other employee, had to be on the payroll for 10 years before qualifying, and then wouldn't be accepted if older than age 59. She would have been 60.

So the competitive offers paled rapidly on closer inspection, thanks in part to the worksheet I provided and helped Joyce fill in. She found that her job at Dr. Neff's was worth $11,700 in salary, you'll recall—but that the salary was only a part of the story. Dr. Neff routinely paid time-and-a-half for overtime, which meant more than $800 a year to Joyce, plus a Christmas bonus equal to one week's base pay.

Also, Joyce participated fully in the practice's retirement plan (Dr. Neff had incorporated). Add to that the health-expense reimbursements, convention expenses, and the premium for her $5,000 of group-term life insurance, and it's easy to see how her benefits package brought her total compensation to $16,564. (Dr. Neff actually budgeted $19,554 for her job, adding $928 in Federal and state employer payroll taxes.) I pointed out to Joyce that the

$3,818 in fringe benefits represented largely tax-free income to her.

Even without considering that tax savings, Joyce saw that she couldn't afford to accept either of the apparently higher-paid jobs offered to her. Her first reaction was disappointment; she'd thought, after all, that she had been offered a way to improve her finances. Her second reaction was more positive. She stopped thinking of her job in terms of the $11,700 base salary and started looking at it as a package worth more than $16,500 in money.

She's much happier now, and she's still working for Dr. Neff.

# 17

# What the professional corporation is really all about

You'd be amazed how many people have the wrong slant on the professional corporation, and I don't mean just doctors. I've heard unbelievable nonsense out of accountants and even lawyers; both should have known the professional corporation cold, right from the start. The problem is that accountants and lawyers sometimes feel it's necessary to deliver any kind of answer other than an honest "I don't know" to any question posed by a client.

But perhaps you won't have as many problems as your senior colleagues encountered, at least not when it comes to the professional corporation. It found its way out into the sunshine back in 1969 through court victories and by weathering a Congressional test of fire late that same year, so it's been around long enough to be within the full grasp now of even the dullest financial advisers. Let us hope.

Since the advisers have had trouble with the concept, don't blame your senior colleagues for not quite getting the point of the professional corporation. One common misunderstanding among them concerns capital and labor. Capital is represented by shares of stock and is rewarded by dividends per share; the dividends bear some relationship to the amount of capital invested. Labor is always conditional on terms of an employment agreement (whether written or oral, specifically detailed or merely implied) and is rewarded with a salary or wages and fringe benefits.

Most medical practices are labor-heavy endeavors, owning relatively little in the way of capital equipment or plant. The exceptions are obvious—radiology, pathology, and any practice that includes, often unwisely, direct ownership of an office building or condominium suite. In the main, though, a medical practice represents very little in the way of capital investment. The value of a medical office lies in its use, rather than its ownership, of equipment and office space.

Since ownership is represented by stock and since a new physician shares in a practice's corporate ownership through the purchase of some of that stock, the difficulty of recruiting a new doctor can be in direct ratio to the expensiveness of the stock. Any practice, small or large, that intends to grow larger one day by bringing in new physicians had better keep the buying-in price as low as possible and not get caught up in the fiction of big financial gains through a new doctor's purchase of the original owner's shares. Far more money will be generated for the practice by an added doctor's services, and financial gains to the doctor he joined will be realized indirectly through the new physician's contribution toward the practice's expenses.

If high valuation of capital stock and resulting discouragement of new physicians who want to join the practice adds up to one problem, an even worse one is the decision to avoid the professional corporation. The principal arguments I've heard against becoming involved with the professional corporation—from here on out, let's call it simply the P.C.—are: "I'm too young," "It's too costly," or "It's too complicated."

Well, there's no such thing as being too young for a P.C.

The principal reason for incorporating is to gain the full rights and benefits of an employee. As we discussed in Chapter 16, a nonincorporated doctor can get some benefits through an I.R.A. or Keogh retirement plan. Much greater gains are possible through a P.C. retirement plan.

The main problem with those last few words is that the term "retirement plan" is usually misunderstood. Forget about all those visions of old age. Starting right now, whenever you hear the words "retirement plan," think of a far more accurate concept: a totally tax-deductible investment program.

To appreciate that definition, you must first comprehend a basic tax truth and the concept of tax-free compounded earnings.

Normally, a reasonably successful investor, physician or otherwise, must earn something like $2,000 after his expenses of doing business and pay something like half of that amount in income taxes in order to have $1,000 left over with which to invest. That's true for any kind of investment—stocks, corporate bonds, municipal bonds, oil wells, real estate, movie deals, or any other kind of investment—*except* a retirement-plan investment. A retirement-plan investment—whether individual retirement account, Keogh, or P.C.—permits investment right off the top—the full $2,000. Further, the retirement-plan investment reduces one's taxable income by the $2,000, thus giving you a lower tax base and, with it, a lower tax obligation. Only investments made to so-called retirement plans permit such tax advantages.

The concept of tax-free compounded earnings involves, first, the number of times those earnings are compounded and, second, the rate of return. To see what that means in terms of a true-to-life situation, consider the typical private practitioner, who, with a typically well-managed practice, shows charges of about $177,200 in 1978, collects about 98 per cent, and banks about $173,650 of gross practice income. He pays about $9,085 for rent and just about $24,000 in employee payroll, plus about $20,600 for other expenses, including malpractice insurance. He takes about $1,300 in reimbursement for professional car expenses and the same for meeting costs; he also gets $3,100 in reimbursement for family health expenses, disability insurance, and term life insurance premiums. His retirement-plan contribution is about $18,000. And his W-2 compensation—salary plus bonuses—totals $83,600.

But never mind the W-2. That $83,600 is a nice living, but the really significant figure is that $18,000 retirement-plan contribution. For illustration's sake, assume that our typical physician never invests more than that amount, despite any continuing increases in productivity and earnings. (Actually, he will invest more, and the additional investment funds will help offset future inflation.) Also, let's assume that he invests $1,500 a month rather than $18,000 at the end of each year. Monthly investment is the best way to go, because of the additional months of investment gained. Let's assume further that he forgoes speculative investments and puts the money into bank savings certificates, bond funds, conservative preferred or common stocks, or anything else that gives a relatively riskless 8 per cent compounded interest.

Working with those assumptions, our somewhat cautious doctor-investor will build up a retirement account totaling $274,400 in just 10 years.

I know. You like your work, and you don't plan to retire in your 40s, even though you're a ripe 35-year-old now. But if you did retire after 10 years, that $274,400, invested at 8 per cent, would yield about $21,950 a year for life. If you wanted to live on some balmy South Pacific island like Paul Gauguin, you could arrange to have the money sent to you in monthly installments—$1,829 a month—which you could probably scrape by on there.

In the real world, you'll keep on working and investing. In 15 years, if you do the same as our illustrative doctor-friend, you should see your retirement account totaling half a million ($519,100); in 20 years, $883,500; in 25 years, $1,426,500.

I won't even tell you what would happen in 30 years. The figure is just too ridiculous to report.

The point is that the longer you get compounded earnings, the better off you are. So the sooner you start, the better for you.

The second excuse for avoiding a P.C.—"It's too costly"—is obviously ridiculous in the face of figures like those. But, of course, not all doctors are typical, nor do they all have well-managed practices, nor do they enjoy typical earnings. The figures I just threw at you were for incorporated general internists. From experience I know that internists fall at just about the midpoint in any statistical study of production and earnings by physicians in private practice. Allergists, cardiologists, and pathologists are often near the top of the gross-practice-income ladder. Pediatricians and psychiatrists are often near the bottom. Those near the bottom of the ladder may need to be concerned about the cost of a P.C. It is more costly, without doubt, than either a partnership or a proprietorship. It will probably become more costly in the future, as the Federal and state governments continue to do what they can to make life more difficult by searching out new ways to tax and by requiring more forms to be filled in for more bureaus, agencies, and departments.

The complaint of complication is valid. The P.C. *is* complicated. Either you can try to unravel the complications yourself, or you can hire someone to do the work for you. The better way is usually to hire someone to do the work, but that isn't always possible. Good professional supportive services are hard to find in many areas, and the cost of bringing in experts from afar, though financially feasible for practices with big numbers, may be well beyond the means of those with only modest gains in sight. Keogh, though also complicated, is comparatively much less so and, more to the point, can be fully administered by mail from afar.

What may be even worse than avoiding the P.C. is playing the P.C. game badly. Poor record keeping, wrong advice, and losing investments can be costly.

If you fail to keep the right records, the Internal Revenue Service may never complain—until you start taking money out of your plan 10 or 20 or 30 years from now. Then you can count on some T-man to do his damnedest to find some administrative gap that will give him an excuse to knock out your plan retroactively and collect taxes all the way back to Day 1. Your alternatives will be to take your financial lumps or to try to beat the I.R.S. in court— spending in legal fees and court costs all the money you thought you'd saved by being your own expert or by hiring inexpert advisers. It's far cheaper to insist on meticulous record keeping and a soundly designed retirement plan right from the start.

Wrong advice can be costly in all sorts of ways, but the kind that allows sloppy or incomplete record keeping or the creation of retirement trust funds that fail to meet the Government's standards is probably the most costly of all. You can't assume that every accountant or lawyer knows everything about everything. It's some comfort, at least, to know that your advisers specialize in P.C. and retirement-trust administration.

Still another blunder to avoid: the wrong kind of investment. There are some pretty good insurance-company plans available, but there are also a lot of bad ones. Some annuities, particularly the investment annuities marketed by insurance companies and by some investment houses and banks, may be all right, depending on the up-front sales commission. What's considerably more punishing is the retirement plan that includes life insurance.

The argument for including life insurance is that the premium is tax-deductible. Well, the tax-deductibility of retirement-plan contributions is only part, probably the least part, of their attraction. That long-term compounded growth we discussed is what puts you into big numbers, and life insurance doesn't grow. Despite the insurance man's terminology, it's not an investment. So the argument that it belongs in a retirement plan is specious, if not downright dishonest.

What's certain is that the insurance salesman will pick up a commission—probably an amount approximating your first year's premium. That's what it's all about.

The loss to you for giving him a payday can be enormous. Since the law allows up to 50 per cent of the retirement-plan contribution to be channeled into life insurance, you can kiss off up to 50 per cent of the growth in your plan. Pick any one of the figures we projected a moment ago, and cut it in half. That's what life insurance could do. And that's expensive.

Now that we've explored some of the opportunities and problems in the P.C., let me add an upbeat thought: In concept, the professional corporation is really not at all difficult. The complexities are connected with the paperwork, and that's easily delegated. Also, the need for the paperwork is easily understood: Federal agencies like the I.R.S. and the Department of Labor require retirement-trust funds to report certain information from time to time so they can see that taxes aren't being underpaid and that the garden-variety employees are getting a fair shake.

To get yourself into a P.C. the right way, you need to take these seven steps:

1. *Get some knowledge.* Medical Economics, Inc., Commerce Clearing House, and Prentice-Hall, among others, have published all kinds of useful and detailed guides to the P.C. You needn't buy them all, but it can help to buy at least a book or two such as "The Whys and Wherefores of Corporate Practice," published by Medical Economics, Inc., Oradell, N.J. 07649.

No book will tell you all you need to know to perform as your own lawyer and trust administrator, but a good book can give you the knowledge you need to decide whether or not to incorporate, select good advisers, and make certain administrative decisions as a good executive should. Figure 17-1 gives you the pertinent addresses, so that you can write for descriptive literature.

2. *Get good start-up documents.* The most important of these documents are the articles of incorporation, the bylaws, and the employment agreement.

You'd be amazed at the number of doctors my management-consulting colleagues have found who have none of those three documents. The absence of any one is enough to prompt an I.R.S. auditor to knock out a P.C. retirement plan, even retroactively, on the grounds that the corporation or its relationship with its key employee (you) is illegal.

The articles of incorporation create the corporation and are filed with the state, usually by mail to the office of the Secretary of State in your state capital. The filing fee is generally modest—for example, it's $61 in New Jersey. The articles, also called the certificate of incorporation or articles of association, specify what the corporation is authorized to do (principally to practice medicine and own property), establish the entity's legality in the state, and establish a contract with the stockholder or stockholders.

The term "professional association" is used in some states—Alabama, Connecticut, Georgia, Illinois, Nevada, New Hampshire, Ohio, Pennsylvania, South Carolina, Tennessee, Texas, and Virginia. The difference between a P.A. and a P.C. is insignificant from a tax standpoint, and both are commonly referred to as professional corporations.

FIGURE 17-1 ═══════════════════════════════════════════

## Some Sources of Help
## for Your Professional Corporation
## and Your Corporate Retirement Plan

Can your lawyer set up your professional corporation and design and provide ongoing administration for your corporate retirement plan? Perhaps. However, the quality of work performed by do-it-all lawyers varies widely, especially in plan design and administration. In my opinion, that's highly specialized work—too specialized to entrust to anyone who doesn't devote full time to it. Some lawyers do just that. Most do not. Anyone who doesn't is probably better off turning to specialists for help, such as those listed below under "Plan design and administration." These books and looseleaf services provide information and advice to you and your lawyer.

☐ Plan design and administration: *Certified Plans, Inc.,* Box 2090, 180 Newport Center Dr., Newport Beach, Calif. 92663; (800) 854-3221

☐ Plan design and administration: PSCC/Profit Sharing Computer Company, 121 East State St., Westport, Conn. 06880; (203) 226-4238

☐ Plan design and administration: Actuarial Services, Inc., 1640 Vaux Hall Rd., Union, N.J. 07083; (201) 686-8686

☐ Book: *The Whys and Wherefores of Corporate Practice,* by Sheldon H. Gorlick, J.D.; Medical Economics Book Division, Inc., Oradell, N.J. 07649; $12

☐ Book: *Now That You've Incorporated,* by Sheldon H. Gorlick, J.D.; Medical Economics Book Division, Inc., Oradell, N.J. 07649; $12.50

☐ Book: *Servicing the Professional Corporation,* by Steven K. Riemer; Prentice-Hall, Inc., Route 59 at Brook Hill Drive, West Nyack, N.Y. 10994; $29.95

☐ Looseleaf: *Corporation Guide,* Prentice-Hall, Inc., Englewood Cliffs, N.J. 07632; $186

☐ Looseleaf: *Professional Corporations Handbook,* Commerce Clearing House, 4025 West Peterson Ave., Chicago, Ill. 60646; $120

☐ Incorporation services to your lawyer: Corporate Services, Inc., 66 White St., New York, N.Y. 10013; (212) 431-5000; corporate filing in 50 states and preparation of all basic documents, seal, etc.; about $50 complete

☐ Referral to plan designers: Conference of Actuaries in Public Practice, 208 South LaSalle St., Chicago, Ill. 60604

The bylaws, which are kept in your office or your lawyer's office, spell out the rules and regulations of the corporation and its stockholders' rights, powers, and duties. The bylaws are to the corporation what the Constitution is to the United States. A corporation without properly drawn and signed bylaws may be attacked as an entity of dubious legality—or of none.

The employment agreement can be merely implied for secretaries, nurses, technicians, and other garden-variety corporate employees, but for safety's sake it needs to be a written agreement for doctor-employees and for any other employees who are shareholders (owners) of the corporation. The employment agreement helps to establish your position as an employee, and it's as an employee that you gain the tax benefits—the right to take part in the retirement plan and so on.

A good employment agreement makes it clear that the patients are those of the corporation, rather than of an individual physician. The distinction is important to the legality of the arrangement. If you're to be an employee of the corporation and thus gain the benefits, you must show evidence to the I.R.S. that you're subject to the control of the corporation. This control is most dramatically exhibited in the corporation's "ownership" of the patients and its right to assign whatever doctor it wishes to any given case.

The articles of incorporation, by the way, also spell out the terms of employment of the doctor-employees, including salary and fringe benefits.

3. *Select the right kind of investment plan.* Your first step is to decide what your investment posture is to be—conservative or aggressive or something in between.

The more aggressive your investment posture is, the more likely you'll need a tailor-made plan that allows the widest possible latitude in the investments you choose. A very conservative plan, on the other hand, may simply lock you into an interest-bearing savings program—a bank's, for instance. The trust agreement for such a plan can be quite simple and inexpensively launched. You may not even need a lawyer; the paperwork can be done by the bank, and a trust office may help you fill in the blanks—the names of your employees, their dates of birth, and the like.

**203**

I'm often asked which investment approach is better—conservative or aggressive. My answer is always the same: The best approach is the one the investor can most easily live with—and that is not a cop-out.

In the retirement-plan example early in this chapter, I assumed an 8 per cent compounded yield—the kind one can easily get these days from investments in corporate bonds, bond mutual funds, preferred stocks, and utility stocks. No such investments are risk-free, to be sure, but none comes close to falling into anyone's definition of high-risk investment. It's even possible to find investment annuities that yield as much as 8 per cent, and some savings banks and savings and loan associations offer term accounts that yield 8 per cent. It's also possible to get a safe 7 per cent from other savings plans and annuities.

Until interest rates tumble, I see no reason whatsoever to settle for less than 7 or 8 per cent, and there's no need for anyone to pay a sales commission for the privilege of earning that much. Banks and no-load mutual funds are happy to write all the savings business they can without charging any sales commission at all.

Make no mistake, though. The difference of even one percentage point can mean a great deal in your investment plan. Look again at our example of $18,000 invested over 25 years. With an 8 per cent yield, the account at the end of 25 years stands at $1,426,500. Drop a full percentage point, and it totals $1,215,100. A million's a million, sure, but the difference here is $211,400, and you can send a lot of grandchildren to college for that.

So just one percentage point makes a big difference. When an 8 per cent yield is as easy to find as a 7 per cent yield, you'd better opt for the 8 per cent.

But what about your older colleagues? Some have set little or nothing aside, and they look forward to only 5 or 10 more years of big earnings. Should they take a flyer?

Answering a question like that is too much like counseling a roulette player to play red or black. Everyone must set his own investment course. Books and essays by the gross have been written on the best way to do so. Some say your investments must stay within the sleep quotient—be no riskier than you can be without losing sleep. So, though it's hard for me to tell anyone he ought to go after more than 7 or 8 per cent these days, I can tell you that many professional portfolio managers claim average annual yields of 12 and 15 per cent. (I said *claim.*) At 15 per cent, that $18,000 yearly investment, in $1,500 monthly installments, produces $132,900 in just five years and $412,800 in just 10 years.

Now, that's spectacular performance. And, though it's the kind of investing that takes me beyond my own sleep quotient, you'll never find me faulting the incorporated doctor who elects to take a flyer—no matter how high. Remember: In a retirement plan, all the growth is totally free of taxes. And that's true even if your investment doubles again and again and again. Only here does our tax system allow so much opportunity to make money.

Once that basic question, conservative or aggressive, has been answered, you're in a position to go out and have the right kind of plan drawn up. Basically, there are two kinds—canned plans, such as those offered by banks, and the customized plans, such as those drawn up by consulting actuaries.

The trouble with trying to find a good consulting actuary to custom-tailor your plan is that most of them sell insurance—and many of them try to conceal that little fact. Unfortunately, there is at this writing no organization of pension actuaries who are wholly independent of insurance interests. There is, though, an organization—Conference of Actuaries in Public Practice, 208 South La-Salle St., Chicago 60604—to which most of the nation's independent actuaries (but also some of the other kind) belong. The organization publishes an annual directory of members, and it will mail you a copy on your written request.

That directory is probably your best printed reference to the expertise you seek. An alternative source is often a medical management consultant, who probably knows of several nearby independent actuaries. And some consultants, largely in a defensive move directly aimed at foiling insurers, have developed retirement-plan design and administration capabilities of their own or can refer you to a selection of law offices with the same capabilities.

Why not just go out and hire a lawyer to design the plan? In theory, any lawyer can do the work, but the fact is that few have the experience. Any lawyer can run down to the law library in the county courthouse and find reference books filled with the boiler plate used in retirement plans, but that's hardly the route to go. For many years, until the mid-1970s, there was seldom any change in pension law. But then all sorts of changes occurred, and so the boiler plate is not always to be trusted. Now the I.R.S. is constantly issuing new rules and regulations, and the person who draws up your plan ought to be someone who does such work full time.

The kind of plan, whether canned or tailored, that you select is as important as any other decision you'll make. For older doctors, a so-called fixed-benefit plan is often the best choice, because the law allows tax-deductible contributions to such a plan in proportion to age. For younger men, a fixed-benefit plan allows a far smaller contribution. So your best bet is almost certainly a combination retirement plan composed of two sections—first, a profit-sharing plan, which permits an annual contribution of an amount equal to as much as 15 per cent of your salary, the amount to be determined by the corporation annually; second, a so-called money-purchase pension plan, which locks you into a predetermined percentage of your salary up to 10 per cent. The total contribution, however, cannot exceed a certain amount set by law. In 1975, the maximum investment was $25,000. But the 1976 Tax Reform Act provided for an annual cost-of-living adjustment to offset continuing inflation. By 1977 the maximum was up to $28,175—a figure announced about April 1 and made retroactive to January 1. Just about any medical management consultant or retirement plan adviser can tell you what the current maximum is.

Now, the good thing about a retirement plan that combines a profit-sharing plan and a pension plan is its flexibility. You've got to make the annual contribution to the pension portion, even if you have to borrow money from the bank to do so, but you have the option of skipping or reducing the profit-sharing plan contribution if you wish. Harking back to our internist with typical 1978 earnings, we find that the combined plan requires an annual contribution of as much as $8,360—10 per cent of his W-2 compensation of $83,600. But he can have his plan written to require a smaller investment. The 10 per cent can be based on his full W-2 compensation (salary plus bonuses) or just on the salary portion alone. If his salary were, say, $30,000, and if his $53,600 in bonuses were exempt, then the pension contribution would be only $3,000.

Unfortunately, many doctors—especially young ones—are opting for the smallest possible contributions, apparently with the mistaken idea that that's the smart route. Well, judge for yourself: $8,360 yearly at 8 per cent becomes $662,500 in 25 years— $424,750 more than $3,000 yearly. *Smart?*

4. *Select solid administration for your investment.* Once your plan has been drawn up, the designer must submit it in your name to the I.R.S. Pension Division for approval.

A prototype plan from a bank, investment house, or other financial institution has already been given I.R.S. approval, and so it needs only a glance from the I.R.S. to see that the information you've entered into the blank spaces passes muster. A custom-tailored plan takes more study, more time. Meantime, you can go ahead and make your first year's contribution. It will be fully tax-deductible if the plan is eventually approved.

It's then, though, that the real problems begin—after all the initial work has been completed. All kinds of reports must be prepared and filed with the Department of Labor and the Department of the Treasury and given to participants and beneficiaries.

The Department of Labor, for instance, requires a Form EBS-1, covering such information as sponsor, administrator, coverage, eligibility, vesting, benefit accruals, claim procedures, identification of fiduciaries, and assignment of plan functions. Also, the Department of Labor requires the filing of Forms 5500, 5500-C, 5500-K, 5500-S Schedule A, and 5500-S Schedule B or 5500-S Schedule C. The same forms—plus Form 966-P, W-2P, 1099R, and W-3—go to the I.R.S. Participants and beneficiaries must receive, by law, a summary plan description, an annual report, tax information returns, written notification of any plan changes, and an annual statement showing total benefits accrued, among other information.

In other words, the continuing administration is no do-it-yourself project.

You need a specialist to handle all that business, and that

doesn't mean just any accountant plucked out of the telephone book. Since the reporting requirements are subject to change at any moment, you've got to make sure that someone who's fully aware of all new developments is doing the paperwork for you. That means an expenditure of time and expertise, and you'll have to pay for it—possibly in the neighborhood of $750 a year.

The main thing to remember is to ask the person or organization designing your plan whether or not he's going to take care of *all* the continuing paperwork, too. If he can't, you may be in big trouble if you let him design the plan. By and large, the people who do provide the continuing administration are reluctant to provide it for any plan other than one they themselves designed.

That's one of the big problems with prototype or canned plans. If the sponsoring organization won't handle the continuing administration, you'll probably end up relying on some accountant down the street, rather than a specialist in plan administration. So much is at stake here—remember those big numbers in our example—that it's foolish to take such a chance.

5. *Consider the secondary benefits—and then reconsider.* Your corporation can set up an employee life-insurance plan that's completely separated from its retirement plan. By separating them, you can buy relatively low-cost yearly renewable term coverage, which gives you just as much insurance protection as any other kind of coverage in any amount that an insurance company will sell you—$100,000, $200,000, $300,000, or more.

At age 30, for example, $300,000 of yearly term insurance costs your corporation a tax-deductible premium of $738, give or take a few bucks, depending on which insurance company you choose. At age 40, the premium, which rises each year, goes to about $1,140 for the $300,000 policy; at age 50, to $2,610; at age 55, to $3,825. Meantime, the tax-sheltered retirement-plan investments keep growing until little or no insurance is needed. When you no longer need life insurance, drop it.

Of course, most insurance salesmen you meet will do their damnedest to talk you into buying whole-life or some other kind of life insurance with cash values. That kind of insurance, as we discussed earlier in this book, costs lots more—even more at age 30 than yearly term insurance costs at age 55. At 30, a $300,000 whole-life policy commands an annual premium on the order of $6,300, and it continues to cost that much every year the insurance is continued in force.

Both kinds of coverage are tax-deductible through the professional corporation—term insurance in an employee life-insurance fringe-benefit plan and whole life in the retirement plan. But, despite all the arguments an insurance man will trot out, term coverage is almost always the better choice. One exception: older doctors who are just starting retirement plans, who can afford to make huge contributions, and who do so by having a fixed-benefit retirement plan drawn up. For them, life insurance—even whole-life coverage—can make sense. But for younger doctors—never.

Also, there's the employee medical plan. Your corporation can establish a plan in which employees are reimbursed for some of their family's health expenses. As we discussed in the last chapter, it's a good idea to set limits on how much an employee will be reimbursed in a year—say, an amount equal to 10 per cent of salary for senior physicians and perhaps smaller percentages for others.

At this writing, there's a question as to the coverage that must legally be provided. One recent major court case held that coverage can be limited to key employees. But most management consultants, including me, recommend that the rank and file be included in the plan, since reimbursement of health expenses costs relatively little and is often highly appreciated by office assistants; it's a useful tool that can help keep the staff happy and productive.

The life-insurance and health-cost reimbursement plans are, in my view, necessities in most practices; I almost always recommend that they be adopted. You don't have to be very imaginative to see what kind of situation you could be in if an employee of yours, particularly one of some tenure and position in the community, dies or becomes totally disabled because of sickness or accident. If the death or disability were not insured, you'd want to contribute something. Well, the best way to contribute is long before any such situation arises, through an employee-benefit plan.

Some other fringe-benefit plans can be included in the package of tax-deductions, but these are of dubious value. Every dollar diverted into a minor fringe benefit is money taken from the amount you could otherwise invest through the retirement plan.

Again, let's put the situation in terms of our typical internist who can put as much as 20 per cent ($17,270) of his total compensation fund of $86,350 into the retirement plan. But if he diverts, say, $6,350 into the minor fringe benefits, he'll be left with $80,000—of which only $16,000 (again, 20 per cent) could be invested through the retirement program. That would leave him with a salary of $64,000.

Many management consultants argue that the indirect price of minor benefits is too high. The difference between $17,270 and $16,000 is $1,270 a year. If invested over 25 years, it could yield $92,800—a stiff price to pay for minor fringe benefits.

Often, your best bet is to participate in the group life-insurance plan but to hold off until the end of the corporate year to decide about taking reimbursement from the health-cost plan. That way, you participate only in a year when your family's health costs really got out of hand.

6. *Make the benefits meaningful to your employees.* Make working for you attractive. A happy staff, motivated by a desire to excel, can make a doctor's professional life highly satisfying.

For instance, look at vesting in the retirement plan. If you wish, you can set up your plan so that no employee fully owns the funds—is vested—until she's been a participant in the plan for a certain number of years. Or, if you wish, she may be vested from the first day of participation. And that, in my very strong opinion, is the only way to go.

Participation can be delayed for, say, a year after the date of employment. That year's delay permits the uncertain and the unsuited employees to come and go quickly without putting you to the expense and bother of enrolling them in the retirement plan and making investments for their accounts. But once an employee— any employee, doctors and nurses and secretaries alike—is a participant, he's also vested.

That's *meaningful* participation.

But knowing what's going on also counts for plenty. All too many medical assistants haven't the foggiest idea what the long-term implications of being in a retirement plan are. It's said that young employees always want cash in the pocket, rather than a retirement plan. If that's so, maybe it's because no one ever took the trouble to tell them about the implications of long-term compounded, tax-free investing.

Suppose a 25-year-old technician who's paid a $7,500 salary has $1,875 invested in her account each year in $156.25 monthly installments. That puts her on a financial track headed directly for $545,500 at age 65. I think you've got to tell employees stuff like that if you hope to gain their enthusiasm for you, your practice, and the job you hope to do for your patients. For half a million dollars, a 25-year-old has good reason to take a strong entrepreneurial interest in your practice. And that's just the attitude you need to encourage. Remember: The first step to financial security for your family is to develop the financial potential of your practice. And you need all the help you can get from your staff.

7. *Don't kill the goose that lays the golden eggs.* Your annual meeting—and you do need to hold an annual meeting of your professional corporation—needs to follow a comprehensive checklist to ensure that all the necessary forms are filled in and all the records are kept and properly filed for the inevitable I.R.S. inspection. Your management consultant or your lawyer—and both of them should be present at the annual meeting—should show up with a printed checklist, rather than try to work from memory.

It's important for a professional corporation to dot every *i* and cross every *t,* even though commercial corporations often don't bother—but then the I.R.S. isn't after *them.* It's long had a thing about professional corporations. The checklist will make sure that you've filed all the tax forms, including those of the retirement plan, and that the book of minutes is completely up to date. Sloppy housekeeping can kill the goose that lays the golden eggs.

Take care, too, that you don't kill it by taking too much out. Many consultants won't fudge when taking deductions for professional-car expenses on the corporate tax return—or for home-office, travel and entertainment, or any other kind of expenses. With hundreds of thousands of dollars at stake in the tax-sheltered retirement plan, it's foolish to chisel nickels and dimes.

**211**

The professional corporation, properly viewed, is a tool that provides access to financial security. Your benefits are obvious. So are the benefits to your assistants. Thus, the P.C. can bring you a secondary benefit by helping create a happy, productive staff.

And there's a big benefit for your patients: Since the P.C. can provide you with solid financial security, you should feel less pressure to raise fees.

For that reason, I truly believe that the P.C. is good—not just for doctors but also for patients. In time, I believe, it will be viewed the same way by Congress and the Federal courts and maybe even by Uncle Sam's tax collector, bless his stubborn bones.

Anything that can bring so much economic security to doctors' families while helping doctors hold the line on patients' health costs is much too important to be entrusted to lawyers and accountants who don't truly know their work. So be sure that your advisers satisfy you that all pertinent tax forms have been filed, that all P.C.-supporting documents are in order, and that their P.C. advice is *informed.* Legal and accounting societies run all kinds of seminars and workshops on P.C.s and pension planning, but not all lawyers and accountants attend—not by a long shot.

If only that were the least of their sins. What bothers me even more is the widespread dishonesty. Supposedly customized retirement plans are actually farmed out by the lawyer to some insurance company's pension department for preparation. The lawyer charges the doctor-client a big fee, although the insurer is actually doing the job free of charge. We've already seen that insurance is made a part of the plan at great hidden cost. And, with or without the insurance taint, many plans are customized so ineptly that they're inferior to some of the canned prototype plans available free or at token expense through banks and investment houses.

If only there were a simple solution, such as hiring a medical management consultant to chair a committee of advisers you know well and trust—a lawyer-buddy, an accountant-friend, you, your spouse. That may, in fact, be your best course, but it's not foolproof. At one time or another I guess every management consultant has himself been skirted or fooled. I sure have. In the end, you pays your money and you takes your chances. Good luck.

# 18

## Productivity:
## Your livelihood depends
## on it

I once tried to attend a three-day national meeting on group practice. I say "tried" because I didn't last through the second morning, and I don't know how I found the patience to sit through the entire first day. Every speaker I heard was from a big prepaid group practice where doctors are paid on straight salary. All but one, as I recall, was an internist, but the lone pediatrician's message was the same as all the internists': "Salaried practice is just terrific because its incentive is qualitative patient care, rather than assembly-line medicine."

I still get ticked off when I think back on that conference.

As I've said before, everyone is paid in either of two ways—in time or in money. It's also true that doctors who think fast and move fast also work fast and are much more productive than doctors who don't do any of those good things—and none of this has a thing to do with assembly-line medicine. It may have a great deal to do, however, with *qualitative* patient care.

**213**

## Getting started in private practice

Anytime I talk about high productivity in a medical office, my underlying assumption is that the people there are able to think fast and well. That's exactly the combination of traits needed in the patient-care segment of medicine. There are in this country more than 215,000,000 patients and not many more than 200,000 M.D.s in full-time private practice—a ratio of 1,075 to 1. Anyone who thinks that an internist should never see more than six or eight patients in a day obviously belongs in salaried practice—like those who, at that seminar, took turns arguing for exactly that kind of patient load.

In the real world, someone's got to tend the sick. They want prompt diagnosis and treatment, and they want to get it in a manner that's somewhat less than offensive.

A great deal of light was shed on those points late in 1976, when Medical Economics published a special issue on patients' attitudes—the result of the largest sampling of patients ever undertaken. To me, the issue was valuable not only for the fresh information presented but also becuase it prompted me to think again about that old term "assembly-line medicine." More than ever, I'm convinced that the complaint usually has very little to do with the amount of time patients are in the office or spend with the doctor. The real complaint is something else—a combination of complaints, really, probably centered on the rushed, even frantic manner displayed by some doctors. Witness these complaints drawn from the questionnaire returns:

> My doctor *races* from one cubicle to the next. . . . He *runs* in and out of doors, speaking *rapidly* and not waiting for any answer. . . . All the time I'm with this doctor, he seems to be doing other things, checking other records, and making calls on the phone—working on me in between. . . . My problems may sometimes sound trivial to him, and he acts that way. But they're important to *me*. . . . Rushed. . . . Bored. . . . Aloof. . . . Impatient. . . . He talked to the nurse the whole time, but not to me. . . . Lack of concern. . . . Hurry up, operate, collect. . . . Snap decisions. . . . Thoughtlessness. . . . I wasn't getting enough information on my medication. . . . They had no time to answer questions. . . . I don't have to pay somebody to be rude to

me. . . . He implied I had a mental problem, but it turned out to be mononucleosis. . . . If he couldn't find the cause, he'd just tell me it was all in my head. . . . I resent being treated as a child or as too dumb to understand. . . . I could more readily accept "average" skill than less-than-average humanism. . . .

One of the fine medical management consultants who reviewed the questionnaires for the magazine and took part in a round-table discussion afterward, Millard K. Mills of Waterloo, Iowa, got right to the nub of the matter, I think, when he said:

"In my experience, there are five questions the most successful doctor answers for the patient in the course of his treatment: 'What's wrong? What caused it? What are you going to do to cure it? How long will it take? How much will it cost?' If the doctor fails to answer these questions, next day the patient calls the nurse and tries to find out."

What's more, the patient feels that he has been rushed, that he has been a victim of assembly-line medicine. The problem has much less to do with time than with manner and style. The problem is, then, one of human relations, of communication.

The questionnaire returns also support that view by pointing up the growth in the number of patients who want to get in and out of the doctor's office just as quickly as possible—especially businessmen, working people in general, young mothers, and young people. Most people—possibly excepting some housewives with no small children, retired persons, and others with time to kill—feel the way I feel. I'm not in a doctor's office because I'm looking for a friend; I want to know what's wrong and the answers to Mills's other four questions, and I want to be treated kindly.

So, saying that you should seek high productivity is not at all the same as saying that you should race about like the Mad Hatter. All I mean to suggest is that you take basic steps like these nine:

1. *Get enough examining rooms.* A dozen years ago, I'd hardly heard of geriatrics. Since then, I've had three clients who specialize in it. The one I'm going to tell you about is the shy type and asked me not to mention his name, so I'll only say he practices in one of the western states where the Rose Bowl is played.

## Getting started in private practice

Incredibly, he was, when I first met him, trying to run his practice in a three-room office—reception room, a room that doubled as a consultation room and examining room, and a third room that doubled as a small lab and examining room. The work load was killing him, he told me, and I didn't wonder. Patients were

FIGURE 18-1 ══════════════════════════════════════════

### Financial Implications

Many doctors' offices book one patient every 15 minutes like clockwork. They do it from habit, without a single questioning thought. Worse than that, many doctors comfortably settle into that routine, passing the time of day with patients and staff to help stretch the time. There's nothing magic, of course, about the number 15. There's much that can be done to fit the scheduling of patients more closely to the time actually needed to diagnose, treat, and check. This worksheet shows the financial implications of increasing productivity in your practice.

| | Example figures | Your figures | Line |
|---|---|---|---|
| **A.** Annual work weeks, less the number of weeks you plan to be absent for vacations, holidays, study, and sickness | 48 | _____ | A |
| **B.** Patient days a week in your practice | 4 | _____ | B |
| **C.** Patient days a year: Multiply Line B by Line A | 192 | _____ | C |
| **D.** Patient hours a day | 6 | _____ | D |
| **E.** Patient hours a year: Multiply Line D by Line C | 1,152 | _____ | E |
| **F.** Number of patients above the present norm who can be seen per hour by increasing productivity | 1 | _____ | F |
| **G.** Patient increase per year: Multiply Line F by Line E | 1,152 | _____ | G |
| **H.** Estimated production increase per patient in fees generated (minimum per patient equal to fee for routine follow-up visit) | $12 | _____ | H |
| **I.** Added annual production: Multiply Line H by Line G | $13,824 | _____ | I |
| **J.** Estimated added cost of seeing each additional patient, over and above normal | | | |

stacked all over the place, and yet the man spent most of his time waiting impatiently for people to undress and dress and clear out so there'd be a room free to see the next patient. That's a hard way to spend the day.

Even so, I had an awfully hard time convincing him to invest

## of a Boost in Productivity

| | Example figures | Your figures | Line |
|---|---|---|---|
| operating costs, including payroll, drugs, supplies, electricity | $1 | _____ | J |
| K. Total annual extra cost: Multiply Line J by Line G | $1,152 | _____ | K |
| L. Fees actually collected: Multiply Line I by your collection ratio: □.96 □._____ | $13,271 | _____ | L |
| M. Net practice income gained from increased productivity: Line L less Line K | $12,119 | _____ | M |
| N. Added amount invested through your corporation's retirement plan: Multiply Line M by □.20 □._____ | $2,423.80 | _____ | N |
| O. Added monthly installment in retirement plan: Line N divided by 12 | $201.98 | _____ | O |
| P. Number of years you will remain in full-time practice—to nearest multiple of 5 | 20 | _____ | P |
| Q. Compound interest factor applicable to Line P: □5:1.4898 □10:182.9460 □15:346.0382 □20:589.0204 □25:951.0263 □30:1490.3594 □35:2293.8824 | 589.0204 | _____ | Q |
| R. Long-range value of increased productivity through retirement plan: Line Q multiplied by Line O | $118,970 | _____ | R |
| S. Long-range value of increased productivity through increased salary: Line M multiplied by .80 [_____] multiplied by Line P | $193,904 | _____ | S |
| T. Total long-range value of increased productivity indicated at Line M: Add Lines R and S | $312,874 | _____ | T |

in a new office for himself—actually, a whole building, even though he was only in solo practice. The new place, only two blocks away from the old and closer to public transportation has—are you ready for this?—11 examining rooms. That's right. For one man. Plus one lab, one X-ray room, one film-filing room with an automatic film processor, a business office, a big reception room, a staff room for meetings and lunches, an audiovisual room equipped with three back-of-screen projectors—one each for filmstrip, glass-mounted slides, and super-8 motion-picture film, all with sound—and three consultation rooms—one for himself and two shared by the various specialists he brings in for half-day turns, rather than sending patients all over town to see them.

Including land, the project cost $110,500 (this was a few years ago), and paying off the mortgage helped to increase the man's overhead by a multiple of four. But his gross practice income also increased by the same multiple, as did his net income—from $40,000 to $160,000 inside 18 months.

That was the doctor who taught me it's easier to get through a highly productive working day than the other kind. The man likes money as well as the next person, but that's not why he's in geriatrics or in that big office. Lots of retired people like to take their sweet time when they visit a doctor's office. *These* retired people are greeted and fussed over and pampered by a smart, capable, friendly, concerned staff of assistants who truly like them and lavish lots of time on them.

The doctor shares their attitude toward the patients, and he makes sure that all five of consultant Mills's mandatory questions are satisfied with *every* patient on *every* visit. He never seems rushed, he listens patiently, his attention is never distracted from the patient, and he never seems to be in a hurry.

But he never wastes time waiting for anyone or anything.

He dictates after seeing each patient—in the patients's presence. Whenever he needs to dictate something that he doesn't want the patient to hear, he adds a postscript on the dictating machine kept at the nursing station.

Most important, he has so many examining rooms that he doesn't care how long it takes a patient to get dressed or undressed.

**218**

He may, for all I know, have more examining rooms than any other solo doctor in the country. But as far as he or his assistants or I know, none of his patients has ever accused him of practicing assembly-line medicine—not since he moved out of the old, cramped office where such complaints were heard.

2. *Question your need for a consultation room.* Look, you'll spend some of the best years of your life in your office, so you've got every right to make it just as comfortable as you like. So you'll hear no complaints from me if you want a room of your own—a consultation room—where you can put your feet up on the desk, read your mail, sign your papers, take a catnap. You might even talk with patients there.

Whether or not it makes sense for you to do so depends on your specialty. When you discover that someone has something seriously wrong and you think it would be more comforting for him to hear the news in your consultation room, rather than in an examining room, then the consultation room is a good choice. It may also be just right for a discussion with several members of a patient's family or in any number of other situations. But, by and large, the consultation room is used too much—and perhaps mainly from habit. Many practices opened in new offices in recent years are doing without that kind of room. Patients don't mind talking in examining rooms, in audiovisual educational rooms, or, when necessary, in the staff lounge/meeting room.

From a doctor's point of view, the best meeting place is usually the examining room. When the discussion is over, he can gracefully take his leave; he needn't be concerned about finding a tactful way to shoo a patient out the door, as he generally must do when the meeting takes place in a consultation room.

So, yes, do question your need for a consultation room, especially when you're starting practice and looking for ways to save space. You'll save some space by doing without, and you won't get into the habit of wasting time behind a desk.

3. *Plan ahead.* When you're starting out, you can get by without an audiovisual room. In fact, in some specialties automated instruction to patients makes little sense. But in some others, an audiovisual room can be useful. For instance, in OB/Gyn, all sorts

**219**

of excellent audiovisual materials are available, as they are in internal medicine, pediatrics, and family practice.

To learn more about the software available, you need only address an inquiry to some of the audiovisual companies in Figure 15-2 in Chapter 15. Also, look for new companies in the patient-education field; they're growing fast, and there's no reason not to expect worthwhile materials from them.

Be alert, too, to the potential of new services, ideas, and equipment of all kinds. Before you move to a new office, you'll need to know what equipment is to go into it, where it's to be located, and how many assistants will be needed to keep it running. That kind of planning ahead can pay off handsomely in higher productivity.

FIGURE 18-2

## Example of an Appointment Day
## That Works

| | |
|---|---|
| 7:30- 8:30 a.m. | Rounds at hospital |
| 9:00-10:00 | Patients who don't mind waiting, such as elderly patients and housewives without kids or jobs |
| 10:00-10:30 | The same, plus sick, injured, and others who can't wait. |
| 10:30-11:30 | Routine scheduling; where possible, bunch patient-types by day or by hour |
| 11:30-11:45 | Catch-up time, drop-ins, emergencies |
| 11:45-12:00 | Telephone call-backs; sign papers |
| 12:00- 1:00 p.m. | Lunch |
| 1:00- 2:00 | Patients who don't mind waiting, such as elderly patients and housewives without kids or jobs |
| 2:00- 2:30 | The same, plus sick, injured, and others who can't wait. |
| 2:30- 4:30 | Routine scheduling; where possible, bunch patient-types by day or by hour |
| 4:30- 4:45 | Catch-up time, drop-ins, emergencies |
| 4:45- 5:00 | Telephone call-backs; sign papers |
| 5:00- 6:30 | Professional reading and other study |

4. *Tailor your appointment system.* There was a time when any doctor who wanted to go on an appointment system had to put in a lot of work selling the idea to patients before they'd begin to accept it. Today, the notion of doing without appointments seems odd. The days of dropping in on people, even doctors, are long gone, and I guess just about everybody knows that.

The problem today is finding or designing an appointment book to fit your particular needs. In Chapter 9, we discussed exactly that point, with special reference to Bibbero's excellent selection of appointment books and Colwell's free kit for customizing an appointment system.

Both of those medical cataloguers, like the others listed in Chapter 9, offer appointment-reminder slips. Your staff should never let a patient get out the door without one unless he's not to be scheduled for another visit. Some charge slips include a section for entering the date and time of the patient's next visit.

There are charge slips, notably Bibbero's, that include a special section for the doctor to indicate the duration of the patient's next visit and approximately when that visit is to occur. But you don't really need a special section on the charge slip to convey such information. By prior arrangement with your staff, you can indicate, say, a five-minute revisit by entering the number "5" on the back of the charge slip, then a slash or a dash, then "2D" or "2W" or "2M" to indicate that the new appointment is to be scheduled in two days or two weeks or two months.

Never, but never, whether in the office or outside it, give a patient a specific day and time for an appointment. That's the job of the appointments secretary or, in the terminology used by some management consultants, the time manager. No matter what the title you give her may be, she will be the most important of all the assistants in your office. She manages your time, so she needs to be a very capable person.

In addition to managing your time, she's also your office's primary contact with the public, so she needs to be an expert at public relations, in dealing with the public, and in handling emergencies and the unexpected. If she's a simpleton, forgetful, or a first sergeant, heaven help you.

In Chapter 9, we also mentioned patient-recall systems, so I don't need to do more than remind you here that the medical cataloguers offer excellent versions and that a recall card, addressed by the patient to himself while in the office, should be mailed about one week before the scheduled appointment whenever more than a month will pass between appointments. Put one person in charge of the recall system, and you'll have every reason to expect the cards to go into the mail on schedule.

It's a good idea, too, to post a sign at your reception window or desk with the request, "Please give 24 hours' notice if you must cancel an appointment." The same message ought to be printed or stamped on recall cards, appointment-reminder slips, monthly statements, and patient-information leaflets. Some management consultants think that patients ought to be charged for breaking appointments without such notice or for not showing up, but I tend to disagree. Well, O.K., a psychoanalyst, to choose one obvious exception, may be justified in making the charge. But most other practitioners are hurt very little by no-shows when they do a good job of advertising that request for 24 hours' notice and if they use both patient-recall cards and reminder slips routinely.

Also, bunching patients by medical complaint or need is a good and time-tested idea. The idea works, several doctor-clients have told me, because they can see one patient after another with just one set of problems in mind. A rhythm is established, and they tend to do a more thorough job in much less time. Infants in for well-baby checks are suited for bunching, as are some other patients—pregnant women, children for school and camp physicals, fatties, and hypertensives, among others. You get the idea.

Your appointment system can even be tailored to cope with the four kinds of patients long identified as major threats to an otherwise orderly office day—the latecomer, the talker, the drop-in, and the emergency.

The persistent latecomer who's coming in for a routine check can be scheduled as the last patient in the day. That way, if he's too late, the door's locked. When he asks to come again, he's given another appointment—same time, another day.

Similarly, the talker can be scheduled as the last patient in the day or as the last patient seen before lunch. Then you can ease him out by telling him that you must get to a luncheon meeting or to the hospital.

On a busy or even on a normal day, the drop-in with a routine problem can be given an appointment for a more suitable day. On a dull day, he can be given a same-day appointment— perhaps in catchup time. That's a 15-minute segment scheduled at least once each half-day in the office, often starting half an hour before lunch or closing time.

An emergency patient whom you know can be scheduled as a drop-in or seen right away if it really is an emergency. If you don't know the patient, you can see him as a drop-in or send him elsewhere when there's a better place to go—the office of a less-busy practitioner, perhaps, or to a hospital's emergency room or outpatient clinic. You've got to be alert to such treatment alternatives for emergency patients, because they, more than any other kind, can make a shambles of your appointment system. Don't routinely accept all emergency patients. Many of them can get good care more quickly elsewhere.

Then, finally, there's the phone. The main thing to remember here is never to take a call if you can call back later. It's a good idea to schedule one 15-minute callback period for each half-day in the office, the last 15 minutes before lunch and the last 15 minutes before closing time.

Figure 18-2 shows a sample appointment day that works.

5. *Never pick up a pencil.* One of the smartest men I've ever met is a management consultant in Norman, Okla., named Roger Harrison, so it's not for nothing that I asked him who's the smartest doctor he'd ever met, and he told me Dr. Orville Rippey of Stillwater. This was years ago, when I was an editor at Medical Economics magazine. I asked Roger if he'd arrange an interview with Dr. Rippey, so I could take a look at his practice and maybe write an article about him and it. He did, and I did.

Dr. Rippey was amazing. He called himself a G.P., but he had a reputation for being as good a diagnostician as any internist I've ever met, and his reputation in OB/Gyn, pediatrics, and anesthesiology was equally good. And on top of all that, the man had no small reputation as a surgeon. But never mind his clinical reputation. What blew my mind was the man's management skills.

When he told me that he tries never to touch a pen or pencil in his office, I guess a puzzled expression came over my face, and so he explained:

"A doctor is like a detective. He puzzles out what's at the root of things. But he's got all kinds of technical help—people to draw blood, do labwork, take X-rays, take patient histories, and all the rest. Very often, I don't even have to talk to a patient before knowing enough about his problem to order the technical work I'll need. In fact, most of the time I order any testing or X-rays even before the patient gets to my office.

"When he does get to my office, he's shown into an examining room by an assistant, and the technical people have their way with him and put their reports in my hands before I ever see him. Then, after I review the reports, I can go further into his history and his complaint. If all that doesn't give me a diagnosis, I probably need more diagnostic work done. Often, we can do that right in my office, because it's very well equipped—especially the lab, which I share with the other doctor-tenant in my building. Or, if necessary, I send the patient across the street to the hospital after phoning across my orders. They generally see him right away and get him right back to me.

"I like being a doctor—especially when I'm a diagnostic detective on a puzzling case. It's a challenge. When a patient gets out of my office without a diagnosis, I've failed. It happens, but we—the people on my staff and at the hospital and I—try not to let it happen.

"I've failed as a manager any time I have to pick up a pencil or a pen for anything other than to sign my name. I'm paid to think, not to scribble. I pay other people to write things for me with pencils and pens and typewriters. Anytime I catch myself doing their work, I realize I'm not doing mine."

When I said something flattering about Dr. Rippey's well-organized approach to practicing medicine, he laughed and said:

"Oh, no, I'm not a well-organized person at all! I'm probably the most disorganized man you've ever met. There was a time when I couldn't cope with the smallest fraction of the patient load I carry now. The patients sitting in the reception room embarrassed me. Why should people have to sit around and wait for me just because I can't get my act together? So, if my practice appears to be well organized, it's for lots of good reasons.

"Mostly, I suppose, it's because I work at it—organization. I hired Roger Harrison the minute I heard about him, and he's been a big help to me.

"He and I worked out the office routine together. When I walk into the office in the morning, I head straight for my consultation room, and the staff follows right in behind me. The office charts have been pulled for all patients scheduled for the day. The charts are stacked on my desk in order—first patient to be seen on top. The nurses have already assigned themselves to various patients so that they can do what's needed in proper order without appearing to be rushed—*ever*. I review each chart quickly. I order diagnostic work done. Since all the charts are in order, it doesn't take long to review them; I can get through the whole stack—often, 40 or so— in less than 10 minutes.

"The staff clinical meeting usually doesn't last any longer than that, and it takes place every morning exactly like that. Everyone then leaves me, except for the office manager, and she and I discuss any administrative matters that need attention. That's her chance to tell me when Roger's coming next, about some staffing problem that appears to be developing, about some new piece of clinical or business equipment that I ought to look into. I try to keep my finger on everything, because it's lots easier and quicker to forestall a problem in the beginning than to try to solve it after it's grown into a monster.

"And I guess you could call me a gadget freak. I'll buy any piece of equipment that will save me a minute. I don't care what it costs. If it saves me a minute an hour, it will pay for itself quickly enough, no matter the price. More important than that, it will help me do a better job for my patients in a more relaxed, better-organized way."

6. *Delegate, delegate, delegate.* Dr. Rippey just told you why a doctor delegates, and, of course, he would, if you asked him, give

you all the caveats. Staff selection, he told me, is all-important. You can't delegate to someone who isn't stable, responsible, understanding, and thoroughly trained.

That's just one reason why you should never hire the cheapest help you can find. Cheap help isn't cheap.

And when you give instructions, make sure they're clear. You haven't delegated a job until your assistant knows exactly

FIGURE 18-3 ═══════════════════════════════════

## What Your Child Can Do

### High-School Level: Some Special Training Required

☐ Take height, weight, pulse, temperature, blood pressure

☐ Prepare examining and treatment rooms for next patients

☐ File ECG tracings

☐ Develop X-ray films

☐ Transcribe chart notes, special reports, referral letters, other correspondence

### Junior-High or High-School Level: Office Training Only

☐ Prepare monthly statements (photocopy or other billing system)

☐ Code ledger cards and insert collection reminders with statements

☐ Get doctor's O.K. and turn accounts over to collector or lawyer

☐ Schedule appointments in routine situations

☐ Maintain the daysheet, making entries and totaling columns

☐ Post the ledger cards

☐ Maintain inventories of office supplies and reorder specified items

☐ Total charge slips and superbills

☐ Prepare routine insurance forms

☐ Maintain records on outstanding insurance claims

☐ Maintain daily and monthly totals on production, adjustments, charges, payments, and key items of expenditure, such as rent and payroll

☐ Write checks

☐ Reconcile checkbook

what you need and want. But you shouldn't let her think that delegating is an invitation to go one step beyond her authority. Medical assistants are technical people, not policymakers. They gather information for you to study. They never diagnose. They never treat. But few are born knowing that. Just by trying to be helpful or trying to do a better job, they can go a step too far. That's the problem and you've got to be able to deal with it. Talk to your

## to Earn Money in Your Office

☐ Prepare daily bank-deposit slip
☐ Prepare monthly Federal and state payroll tax forms
☐ Maintain payroll records
☐ Prepare annual W-2 forms in January or when an employee leaves
☐ File office charts; pull charts for incoming patients
☐ Transfer inactive charts to storage
☐ Microfilm inactive charts
☐ Maintain referral records

### Grade-School or Junior-High Level: Minimal Training Needed

☐ Pick up messages from answering service or machine
☐ Photocopy and distribute day's appointment sheet
☐ Register new patients
☐ Turn on office lights and sound system, make coffee, adjust thermostat
☐ Get, sort, distribute mail; count and endorse checks received
☐ Post outgoing mail, turn off sound system and lights, adjust thermostat
☐ Water the office plants
☐ Sterilize instruments
☐ Clean bathrooms; restock paper towels, cups
☐ Empty wastebaskets; vacuum; mop, wax, dust, polish; carry trash to curb
☐ Wash windows, mow lawn, trim shrubs, shovel snow
☐ Run errands

office assistants. Be sure to tell them just what they need to be told.

Supervise closely, as Dr. Rippey does. Then you'll automatically be checking on performance.

What kind of tasks should you delegate? Almost every task related to the gathering of information and short of making a clinical decision.

In various specialty practices, appropriately trained medical assistants and physician's assistants are doing well-baby exams; administering psychological tests; performing psychiatric social work; applying and removing casts; obtaining electrocardiograms and electroencephalograms; doing refractions, tonometry and muscle-balance determinations; doing routine deliveries; and giving instruction to patients, often in conjunction with audiovisual programs on diet, obesity, child care, eye care and contact lenses, preoperative and postoperative care, hospitalization planning, special medication, birth control, and prenatal and postpartum care. In general and specialty practices alike, a whole list of duties are often delegated. Some of them can be handled even by children, as you see in Figure 18-3.

7. *Set a reasonable budget for personnel.* In the first three years or so of your practice, your time will be worth from $25 to $70 an hour, not counting time spent in travel and continuing education and otherwise not directly involved with patient care.

Even if you make only $25 an hour, that's a lot more than you'll be paying your assistants. There's no point in your doing $7.20-an-hour work when you can be doing $25-an-hour work for patients, is there? But $7.20 is the hourly rate of a 40-hour-a-week, $15,000-a-year employee, and I'll bet you're a long way off from paying that much. You get a $12,000 employee for $5.76 an hour, a $9,000 employee for $4.32 an hour, a $6,000 employee for $2.88 an hour.

That's why doctors—and management consultants, businessmen, and executives—delegate. And that's why you need to hire a staff.

As your practice grows, as you become more productive, and as you work smarter, rather than harder, your hourly production rate will rise, and your need for more help will expand. That's one of the big reasons why you'll be wise to get all the figures you need, right from the very first month of practice, for the monthly management report you'll find in Chapter 20.

As production increases, there's an automatic need to increase the payroll budget. Sometimes, as when growth is slow, the increase will be reflected mainly in pay raises to competent assistants whose capabilities increase meritoriously. Never overlook the pay raise as a means of keeping competent help.

Figure 19-3, in the next chapter, is a table showing typical medical-office staffing figures by specialty. So there's no need to go into great detail here, but a rough rule of thumb covering all specialty practices couldn't hurt, could it? Here you go:

Annual production multiplied by .0083 gives a minimal budget for medical-office staffing in many practices; multiply production by .0125 for a middle-of-the-road budget; multiply by .0183 for an aggressive budget in a rapidly growing practice. That formula—again, it's just a rough guide—gives a *monthly* payroll budget. If you're used to thinking in terms of weekly pay, multiply production by .0019, .0029, and .0043.

8. *Set a reasonable budget for office space and equipment.* We've talked about the importance of a well-designed office in the quest for a productive practice that's pleasing to patients, doctors, and staff. But there's another basic ingredient, and that's equipment—clinical and business.

That, too, is covered in detail in the next chapter, and Figure 8-1 in Chapter 8 provides a special worksheet. It reflects my rule of thumb: Any doctor will be office-poor if he pays more than 9.5 per cent of his projected production for office space and equipment, but just about any doctor with a growing practice can afford to budget 9.5 per cent.

9. *Get all the diagnostic tools you need.* The key word in that sentence is "need." Tools you don't really need are toys, though perhaps convenient and tempting. Wait till you're a superstar to buy clinical equipment that makes little sense economically.

In time, you may be like the radiologist-client of mine who once spent $75,000 on an exotic machine that he uses perhaps once every six months—not because he needed it but because he'd heard that a crosstown rival had just bought the same thing. As it turned out, the rival hadn't; it was just a false rumor, started by some wag in the doctors' lounge. But when the rival heard about my client's purchase, he did, in fact, order the same machine.

Perhaps I should add that you should get all the diagnostic tools you need *when* you need them. All too often, the doctor new in practice overextends himself in one area and makes up for it by scrimping in another. The area of overextension is often clinical equipment. It may be tough doing without all the tools you had at your command while in training, but, unless you're already rich, you'll have to set realistic priorities.

And then there's business-office equipment. But that subject is a chapter all by itself—the next one.

# 19

## Productivity:
## Your business office
## needs it, too

The work to be done in your business office couldn't be more vital to the successful and continuing operation of your practice. You need to keep that in mind always. Words must be processed. Financial record keeping and billing must be done. And the business office is the site and source of virtually all information needed to support such key management decisions as the expansion of the office or its staff and the recruiting of an additional doctor.

To cope with those tasks, you need not only staff but tools—things made of metal, plastic, and glass, yes, but also concepts reduced to worksheets or other kinds of forms—clinical records and monthly management reports, for instance.

If you trained in a hospital with a highly automated records system, you may be far more turned on by the idea of a computer-assisted medical practice than many of your senior colleagues ever will be. Several excellent hospital systems have been in use for several years now, and they handle clinical, financial, and management information with varying degrees of simplicity and capability. The Technicon, Inc., system installed in Bethesda by the National Institutes of Health is perhaps foremost in the handling of information. The system consists of a large central computer tied in with minicomputers and accompanying cathode-ray tube terminals for videoscreen display. Sophisticated and costly as it is, even that system or one much like it may well find its way into your office someday—not the big computer but the minicomputer and terminal. Your equipment will be linked by phone or telegraph wire to a central computer at your group practice's business office, hospital foundation for medical care, health-maintenance organization, county medical society, or elsewhere.

In time, perhaps in five years or so, the memory capability of your office minicomputer will be equal to that of some of the largest computers on the market today. The capacity of the central computer to which it will be linked will be correspondingly greater. Access will usually be instantaneous, and, as a result, you won't bother keeping paper records in your office anymore.

The capability is here right now. Capability isn't the problem. Cost is the problem. The computer industry, as most know it today, owes its life to the transistor, which replaced the tube. In turn, the transistor is being replaced by the almost incredible silicone chip. Even more incredible devices are just around the corner. So computers, like pocket calculators, will get smaller and less costly.

The day isn't far off when children—certainly your grandchildren and probably *your* children—will be amazed when told that people actually used to live in houses without computerized TV sets to aid them with shopping, letter writing, access to all the information once deposited in all the libraries of the world, taxes, opinion sampling, voting, and homework. Or that doctors' offices managed somehow to blunder along without the same kinds of terminals to provide computer-assisted diagnoses and treatment indications and to do all the record keeping and filing. There's a good chance that in the near future a terminal and its operator will handle all the traditional front-office chores of half a dozen doctors—and do it in a six-hour working day.

Back in the real world of today, the computer has limited

application in a private medical office. Computer-prepared billing and insurance-form preparation can be worthwhile, especially when the accompanying management reports are truly useful—for instance, when keeping all the data required for a completely fair, productivity-based compensation system in a multidoctor practice. And you needn't buy a computer to enjoy its use; that's why medical computer-billing companies exist.

Until inexpensive terminals and associated systems are available, you need to give careful consideration to all the traditional equipment and systems—especially those related to clinical record keeping. As mentioned in Chapter 9, some medical cataloguers offer good, basic clinical-record systems, and you ought to review them to see if they fit your needs when you open shop. But more sophisticated systems also demand your attention. Lots of people have devoted time and thought to the design of better clinical-record systems printed on paper. Many of these people are members of the American Medical Record Association, 875 North Michigan Ave., Chicago 60611.

A number of attempts have been made with varying degrees of success to design clinical-record forms that require more checking of boxes and less writing or dictating—and for good reason. It can cost a small fortune to have all your office charts transcribed and typed. The goal is detail and clarity comparable to a typed chart—but in a simple, hand-prepared chart.

The best attempt I've seen to date is a system of problem-oriented medical records created by Lawrence L. Weed, M.D., and today sold by Shingles, Inc., in a streamlined version modified for use in a busy private office. The early Weed version was designed for use in hospitals and teaching. The new version costs about 30 cents per patient for start-up and 10 cents per patient yearly for continuing use. The system includes 16 different forms, 100 to a pad, at $2.40 a pad.

Another highly sophisticated paper system is sold by Patient Care Systems, Inc. A third system is sold by Bibbero Systems, Inc. You may want to compare those three systems, along with any similar systems you find, before making a choice.

*(Continued on page 236)*

FIGURE 19-1 ═══════════════════════════════════════

## Some Sources of

### ASSISTANT TRAINING AND PATIENT EDUCATION

☐ Bell & Howell, Audio-Visual Products Division, 7100 North McCormack Rd., Chicago, Ill. 60645; (312) 262-1600

☐ Dukane Corporation, Audio-Visual Division, 2900 Dukane Dr., St. Charles, Ill. 60174; (312) 584-2300

☐ Eastman Kodak Co., 343 State St., Rochester, N.Y. 14560; (716) 325-2000

☐ Singer Education Systems, 3750 Monroe Ave., Rochester, N.Y. 14630; (716) 586-2020

### COPIERS

☐ Canon, Nevada Dr., Lake Success, L.I., N.Y. 11040; (516) 488-6700

☐ IBM Corporation, Parson's Pond Dr., Franklin Lakes, N.J. 07417; (201) 848-1900

☐ Savin Business Machines Corp., 475 Park Avenue So., New York, N.Y. 19916; (212) 679-2200

☐ Saxon-Scott Copy Machines, 13900 N.W. 57th St., Miami Lakes, Fla. 33014; (305) 822-0500

### DICTATING EQUIPMENT

☐ Craig Corporation, 921 West Artesia Blvd., P.O. Box 5664, Compton, Calif. 90220; (213) 537-1233

☐ Dictaphone, 120 Old Post Rd., Rye, N.Y. 10580; (914) 967-7300

☐ IBM Corporation, Parson's Pond Dr., Franklin Lakes, N.J. 07417; (201) 848-1900

☐ Lanier Business Products, 1700 Chantilly Dr., N.E., Atlanta, Ga. 30324; (404) 321-0911

☐ Lexicon Inc., 60 Turner St., Waltham, Mass. 02154; (617) 891-6790

☐ Norelco, 175 Froehlich Farm Blvd., Woodbury, N.Y. 11797; (516) 921-9310

☐ Sankyo Seiki (America) Inc., 149 Fifth Ave., New York, N.Y. 10010; (212) 260-0200

☐ Sanyo, 1200 W. Artesia Blvd., Compton, Calif. 90220; (213) 537-5830

☐ Sony Corporation of America, 9 West 57th St., New York, N.Y. 10019; (212) 371-5800

## Good Office Equipment

### FILING EQUIPMENT

☐ Dolin Metal Products, Inc., 475 President St., Brooklyn, N.Y. 11215; (212) 596-1400

☐ Eastman Kodak Co., 343 State St., Rochester, N.Y. 14560; (716) 325-2000

☐ Lundia Myers Industries, Inc., 600 Capitol Way, Jacksonville, Ill. 62650; (217) 243-8585

☐ Medical Data Systems Corp., 24541 Bagley Rd., Olmsted Falls, Ohio 44138; (216) 234-9580 (Computer)

☐ Powers Regulator Co., 3400 Oakton St., Skokie, Ill. 60076; (312) 673-6700

☐ Supreme Equipment & Systems Corp., 170 53rd St., Brooklyn, N.Y. 11232; (212) 492-7777

☐ Tab Products Co., 269 Hanover, Palo Alto, Calif. 94300; (415) 493-5790

### TELEPHONE EQUIPMENT

☐ Candela Electronics, 946 Benicia Way, Sunnyvale, Calif. 94086; (408) 738-3800

☐ Executone Inc., 29-10 Thomson Ave., Long Island City, New York, N.Y. 11101; (212) 392-4800

☐ Gimix Inc., 1337 West 37th St., Chicago, Ill. 60609; (312) 927-5510

☐ Pacesetter Communication Corp., 43 West 24th St., New York, N.Y. 10010; (212) 691-6700

### TYPEWRITERS

☐ Adler Business Machines Inc., 1600 Route 22, Union, N.J. 07803; (201) 964-3200

☐ Facit-Odhner Inc., 66 Field Point Rd., Greenwich, Conn. 06830; (203) 622-9150

☐ Hermes Business Machines, 1900 Lower Rd., Linden, N.J. 07036; (201) 574-0300

☐ IBM Corporation, Parson's Pond Dr., Franklin Lakes, N.J. 07417; (201) 848-1900

## Getting started in private practice

Keeping up to date with new developments in clinical and business systems and equipment isn't easy, since changes occur rapidly. Publications like Patient Care and Medical Economics help a lot, for they report on such developments from time to time. Outside the medical publishing field, one especially useful source of information on new business-office equipment is a trade publication called Office Products News, P.O. Box 619, Garden City, N.Y. 11530. The yearly subscription rate of $7.50 is a small price to pay for help in keeping informed about the best buys among the following 14 kinds of office equipment:

1. *Adding machines.* A couple of years ago the Olivetti Quanta T was, in my opinion, the best buy on the market at $115. It's still a good machine, and I recently saw it advertised by an office-equipment discount house in New Jersey for less.

The same ad (in The New York Times) showed the reason why I no longer recommend the Olivetti or any other adding machine: Printing calculators, which do the same work and more, have dropped so much in price that there's no point in buying a machine that only adds. The ad offered a Sharp printing calculator for exactly the same price as the Olivetti adding machine.

Notice that I said a *printing* calculator—the kind with a paper tape, unlike the electronic visual display feature found on your pocket calculator. The paper tape is important, I believe. At the end of each office day, your financial secretary needs to add up the daysheet columns for production, adjustments, charges, and payments, and she needs to do so on a machine with a paper tape so that she can attach the tape to the daysheet for later review by you, your accountant, or your medical management consultant.

2. *Medical-assistant training equipment.* With a Kodak Ektagraphic Visualmaker ($140 at this writing), you or your management consultant can make color slides from books, charts, graphs, ledger cards, magazines, whatever. By using your own cassette tape recorder for vocal instruction and a sound-slide projector like Singer's Caramate II Model 8866 ($449.50 at this writing), you can synchronize sound to slide and create your own on-the-job automated instruction in such tasks as financial record keeping, preparing health-insurance claim forms, and dealing with patients.

Bell & Howell also makes equipment of special interest to anyone interested in preparing such material.

3. *Calculators.* The prices of calculators have dropped so much that today you can buy a pocket version for about 0.007 per cent of the price of a sophisticated desktop calculator available just 10 years ago. That's for a calculator with visual display. Ten years ago, you couldn't buy a printing calculator at any cost. That kind came along a few years later, and it was generally sold in a price range of $350 to $1,200, which was considered terrific. Today, you often see printing calculators advertised in display ads in The Wall Street Journal for less than $100.

4. *Computers.* In a small medical office, or even in a medium-sized one, a big computer by today's standards is completely out of the question. It's too expensive. A minicomputer may be worth considering, depending on the price you must pay for what the machine will accomplish. A mere terminal—with a modified typewriter keyboard and cathode-ray tube for visual display and maybe with a printer hooked to it—figures to cost less.

The brand name of the equipment you use means almost nothing. You need to know what it can do. Even the brand name of the central computer to which the terminal is linked by phone or telegraph wire or, soon, by laser beam doesn't mean a thing. For that matter, the terminal of the future that's best for small offices may be manufactured by a company not even in business today. And the alternative minicomputer may be pieced together from bits and pieces and hunks of hardware manufactured by a number of different companies.

IBM is probably the best-known name in computers. But, big as that company is in maxicomputers, it's small potatoes in the minicomputer and terminal fields. Those two fields have scarcely been opened. You can watch Office Products News for new developments in the months and years immediately ahead.

So many little firms are hard at work on sophisticated minicomputers systems that it's virtually impossible to know what's currently on the market, much less what's coming on the market tomorrow morning or what the best of the new machines is. But among the best are the hardware and accompanying programs

FIGURE 19-2 ═══════════════════════════════════════

## Where to Buy
## Office Equipment Cheaply

Office-equipment discount outlets are to be found in major cities everywhere. Watch for their advertising in daily newspapers—local, regional, and national. Two national publications, The Wall Street Journal and The New York Times, often carry discounters' display ads. Some outlets carry a wide selection of equipment; others are specialized. Some deal mostly by mail order.

If you need a specific item for your office, consider hunting among the more likely discounters for the lowest bid. With the help of a photocopier—your own or the hospital's—run off copies of a form letter that specifies the make and model number of the item you need, asks for a bid that includes shipping price and sales taxes, and sets a deadline date (give them a couple of weeks to respond).

First, though, add discounters of your own discovery to this list:

☐ Accurate Business Machines, 6621 Biscayne Blvd., Miami, Fla. 33152 (CG)

☐ ADM Business Machines, 20 West 23 St., New York, N.Y. 10010 (CGT)

☐ Alpha Business Machine Corp., 300 Fifth Ave., New York, N.Y. 10001 (YCDPG)

☐ American Typewriter Co., 155 North Dean St., Englewood, N.J. 07631 (Y)

☐ Chafitz, 856 Rockville Pike, Rockville, Md. 20852 (C)

☐ Dixie Hi-Fi, 2040 Thalbro St., Richmond, Va. 23230 (DA)

☐ 47th Street Photo, 67 West 47th St., New York, N.Y. 10036 (AD)

☐ Jems Sounds Ltd., 785 Lexington Ave., New York, N.Y. 10021 (DA)

☐ Julor Discount, 1178 Broadway, New York, N.Y. 10001 (C)

☐ Longacre Office Machines, 20 East 40th St., New York, N.Y. 10016 (CT)

☐ Phone Control Systems, 92 Marcus Ave., New Hyde Park, N.Y. 11040 (N)

☐ RCI Discount Appliances, 210 East 86th St., New York, N.Y. 10028 (CG)

☐ Taft Electronics, 68 West 45th St., New York, N.Y. 10036 (D)

☐ Wolff Office Equipment, 1841 Broadway, New York, N.Y. 10023 (T)

☐ Harry Strauss & Sons, Inc., 429 Jersey Ave., New Brunswick, N.J. 08903 (C)

☐ Barco Business Equipment Corp., 44 West 44th St., New York, N.Y. 10036 (DNTG)

☐ Comet Office Products Center, Inc., 99 Madison Ave., New York, N.Y. 10016 (P)

☐ Grand Com Inc., 1152 Sixth Ave., New York, N.Y. 10036 (N)

☐ JS&A National Sales Group, 1 JS&A Plaza, Northbrook, Ill. 60062 (CD)

☐ Willoughby Peerless, 43rd St. and Lexington Ave., New York, N.Y. 10017 (CDAN); 116 West 32nd St., New York, N.Y. 10001 (P)

Key: **A:** audio-visual. **C:** calculators. **D:** dictating. **G:** general. **N:** phone and answering machines. **P:** photocopiers. **T:** typewriters (new). **Y:** typewriters (reconditioned).

offered by Edelman Systems, Inc. They're at least good enough to require comparison to any other minicomputer medical-office system on the market.

The traditional caveat for bookkeeping machines also applies to minicomputers and terminals: You've got to have at least three people in your office trained to run the things. That's not to say that the training period is necessarily long or difficult for every piece of equipment coming on the market. But it sure is saying that you've got to have a regular operator, a No. 2 to take her place when she's on vacation or out sick, and a No. 3 to back up No. 2.

5. *Dictating and transcribing machines.* Almost all dictation used to be on magnetic wires, disks, and belts, but today very little of it is. The standard mechanism today is the audiocassette—a C-60, the same kind that many people buy prerecorded now.

In recent years, the brand names favored by many of the medical management consultants have included Craig, Dictaphone, IBM, Lanier, Norelco, Sony, Stenorette, and Stuzzi. The various dictating units sold under those brand names have a wide range of features, but the value of many of them is suspect.

For years, I used as a dictating machine a $39.95 cassette recorder purchased over the counter at Sam Goody's, a big New York audio and record chain. About a year ago, I replaced it with a smaller Sony TC-55, which costs more than three times as much but is more portable and works off both AC and DC. The accompanying battery pack brought the total price to something like $160.

The list price for cassette recorders means less than it does for other equipment, which is why I'm not going to be very precise here. If you get in the habit of watching for office-machine ads in your local paper and in the national papers (The Wall Street Journal and The New York Times), you discover that you can buy all kinds of equipment well under list price. I have in front of me now, for instance, an ad for an excellent transcriber, a Craig 2706A, for just $179.95, which is something like a third of the usual list price for transcribing machines.

There's a difference between dictating and transcribing equipment. You can get away with an inexpensive cassette recorder for dictating purposes. You start the thing going and speak just as if you were dictating to a stenographer; you don't really need to have the fancy features—indexin_ erasing, whatever—that are added to the more expensive kinds of recorders called dictating instruments. If you change your mind, just say to the recorder, "I changed my mind.' The secretary who transcribes the tape shouldn't attempt to take a finished letter or report off the machine; she should simply do a rough draft. Doing that, she can do whatever she'd normally do if you changed your mind while she was taking shorthand in your presence.

The transcribing instrument is another matter. The basic difference between a dictating machine and a transcribing instrument is that the transcriber has a floor switch to make it go, stop, and back up, but a tape recorder does not. The floor switch allows the secretary to keep her hands on the typewriter keyboard.

Some transcribing machines also have a very useful telephone feature added. After hours, you can phone the line to which your transcriber is hooked up in your office and dictate. That feature alone, to many doctors, makes the transcribing machine a worthwhile investment.

6. *Filing equipment.* Until you get involved with computerized chart filing, your best bet is an investment in shelf filing equipment, such as that sold by Dolan Metal Products, Inc.; Lundia Myers Industries, Inc.; Powers Regulator Co.; S.F.I., Inc.; Snead Manufacturing Co.; Supreme Equipment & Systems Corp.; and, my old favorite, Tab Products Company.

It's important for you to know the difference between shelf filing and the push-pull kind. With shelf filing, you pull or push nothing. The steel filing unit, either with doors or without, does nothing; it just stands there, usually six shelves high, waiting for a chart secretary to put charts there or to file records there. It works like a charm, saves space, and is cheaper than the other kind.

The traditional four-drawer, push-pull filing unit has four drawers because it can't be much higher, since you can file only as high as you can look into. Tall secretaries can, on special order, get five-drawer push-pull cabinets, but why? The moving parts cost extra, and shelf files six tiers high hold more records per square foot of floor space.

## Productivity: Your business office needs it, too

For record storage, there's an increasing trend toward the microfilming of old charts. But buying your own microfilm camera probably isn't a good idea, except maybe for very big practices. Doctors in small practices can always check the Yellow Pages for centralized microfilming services. Their fees have become more competitive in recent years—another example of falling prices in the equipment field—and they can get rid of a lot of paper in your office for something like $18 a thousand images.

7. *Furnishings.* You almost never saw carpeting on the floor of a medical office 10 or 15 years ago. Then people began catching on to the fact that carpeting helps deaden sound and provides insulation. And it often cuts down on the breakage of things dropped in the lab. So plan to get some inexpensive carpeting.

To give you a rough idea of how much you need to spend on cheap furnishings, not decorator items: $24 each for upholstered stacking chairs without arms (they're O.K. while you're starting up your career and are more interested in saving bucks than in looking good; by the time the things fall apart, and they will, you'll be able to afford better); a secretarial desk with a machine extension for a typewriter, $229; accompanying secretarial chair, $60; a 72-inch executive desk (nice) and matching credenza, $675 for the pair; accompanying executive-type chair, $100.

8. *Intercoms.* In most offices the intercom is used mainly to notify someone that he's wanted on the phone. For that kind of conversation, use an intercom built into the telephone system.

Ma Bell provides it on request, so ask for the intercom feature when ordering your phones. But consider the equipment offered by Ma Bell's competitors before you order anything.

Executone is a well-established maker of intercom equipment that now offers excellent telephone equipment—some with features that the phone company doesn't even offer. And, of course, companies like Executone build intercom features right into their phone equipment.

Check it all out. Nowadays there's new equipment being marketed all the time, so I won't try to review what's new here.

9. *Postage meters.* I used to be against the things, because just about the only time they may be needed is on billing day, and

you can buy stamped envelopes from your local post office. But in the past few years, first-class postage rates have changed so often that I've seen many doctors get stuck with envelopes prestamped with the wrong amount of postage, and there's certainly nothing efficient about that.

On the other hand, you can buy a Stamp E-Z—a paper-stamp affixing machine—from a medical cataloguer for lots less than a postage meter costs.

So I have practically no opinion now about a postage machine. In the early, struggling year or years of private practice, you can certainly live without one. Later, it may be a convenience.

FIGURE 19-3 ════════════════════════════════════

## Well-Established Practices Budget
## Up to 21 Per Cent for Assistant Payroll

| Specialty | % of Charges |
|---|---|
| Allergy | 16.8 |
| Anesthesiology | 18.5 |
| Cardiology | 18.2 |
| Dermatology | 15.9 |
| Gastroenterology | 9.0 |
| General and family practice | 16.3 |
| General surgery | 10.4 |
| Internal medicine | 13.5 |
| Neurology | 11.4 |
| Neurosurgery | 11.7 |
| OBGyn | 12.5 |
| Ophthalmology | 13.5 |
| Orthopaedic surgery | 12.7 |
| Otolaryngology | 12.3 |
| Pathology | 21.2 |
| Pediatrics | 14.9 |
| Plastic surgery | 8.0 |
| Psychiatry | 13.9 |
| Radiology | 9.0 |
| Thoracic surgery | 8.8 |
| Urology | 9.7 |

Source: Society of Professional Business Consultants, Chicago, Ill.

10. *Photocopiers.* This field probably bears more watching than any other, since so many new machines are coming on the market now. For your purposes, IBM, Kodak, and Xerox are probably not your best bets. You can pay a lot less for some other brand of bond copier—a Savin, for instance. Those big-name photocopiers cost about $700 a month to lease while the small-name copiers cost about $150 a month.

You pay less for an electrostatic copier. This type comes in two versions—one with liquid toner, the other with powder. The first kind is less costly to buy and produces a coated copy that's hard to write on with a ball-point pen. The second kind is more costly and somewhat easier to write on. The kind of electrostatic copier I've often recommended for use in photocopy billing over the past 10 years or so is still an excellent machine. It has an automatic feeding device that makes billing day a snap. Some 10 years ago it cost $1,200. Now it's priced at $1,900, and I don't recommend it much anymore. Bond copiers—even the kind with automatic feeding devices that shove the ledger cards through on billing day—are worth the extra price, considering the five or more years of daily use you can expect from them and the big savings they yield in lower operating costs.

To purchase a bond copier with IBM-Kodak-Xerox copying quality, you'll probably pay from $3,000 to much, much more through the balance of the 1970s. It's harder to generalize about the future prices of the electrostatic copiers. In the face of all the new competition from the bond copiers, you'd think the inferior electrostatics would be tumbling in price. But so far it hasn't happened—not, at least, with machines that make billing easy.

The best choice for a doctor just starting out may be to select a billing system that needs no copier and to use carbon paper or carbon sets with correspondence, just as everyone did before the photocopier was invented. The alternative billing systems are discussed in Chapter 11. After a couple of years of getting by, you may find that the copier market has settled down and that good buys are as abundant as the selection of good machines.

11. *Security equipment.* This is another volatile area just now, and if you're a gadget freak, pay close attention here. Just

imagine: Rockwell International now offers a Printrak 250 system straight out of Mission Impossible—a system that reads visitors' fingerprints. And Rusco Electronic Cassette Systems does away with the old-fashioned door key by scanning a credit-card-type ID that's virtually impossible to duplicate. It's useful for ensuring that only the right people open doors, cabinets, or parking-lot gates.

In the real world of small business, you can find more security devices than you'll ever need in the free catalogue offered by Mountain West Alarm, 4215 North 16th St., Phoenix, Ariz. 85016. The catalogue lists residential and commercial burglar alarms, closed-circuit TV, silent phone-line connections, and burglar detectors of every description.

Actually, the value of burglar alarms has not yet been conclusively established. They don't seem to scare burglars away, though that's a hard feature to measure. But they do result in the arrest of burglars while still on the premises.

Simpler, more obvious factors may be even more useful than alarms in keeping burglars away. Many burglaries are committed by nonprofessionals—kids, drug addicts. They tend to hit the easiest targets. So an office with well-lit windows and doorways and employees who always remember to lock up when they leave is safer than the other kind.

Should you practice where crime is nonexistent? Forget it. The burglary rates in medium-sized cities are now about the same or even a little higher than those in large cities. So I'm not sure it matters where you practice, as long as it's not in a combat zone. These days, even farmers are seriously concerned about house burglaries and tractor thefts.

Good lighting and locked doors are the mandatory basics everywhere. Anything you do after that may come under the heading of religion.

12. *Sound equipment.* If you're a hi-fi fan, there's no reason why you can't apply your knowledge to your medical office. If you're not, get a reasonably good FM radio and keep it tuned— low—to the local good-music station.

Beware of taped-music systems. It's almost impossible to buy a large enough selection of tapes to keep yourself and your staff from going crazy from hearing the same stuff over and over again.

13. *Telephones.* This field may be even more volatile than photocopying. Years and years of litigation have broken the monopoly of Ma Bell, and new companies by the dozens have swung into the phone-gadgetry market. Ma Bell is responding by coming out with all kinds of new gadgetry of her own.

So now you can buy cordless phones and phones that divert calls from your office to your home phone or to an employee's number. For doctors, that's probably the most significant of the new features since many physicians have been unable to find competent answering services. A call diverter allows assistants to take turns answering the phone off-hours at home.

Also, there's a gadget that links an answering machine to a call diverter. The message on the machine tells a patient to stay on the line for 45 seconds, or whatever, if there's a medical emergency; after that time, the call diverter goes into action if the patient's still on the line.

Answering machines like the Record-a-Call offer two other features: You or your assistant can retrieve messages from the machine by phoning in and using a special remote key, and you can change the message recorded on the machine.

14. *Typewriters.* Typewriters are also being computerized, but you can forget about that until your practice is well established. Automated typewriters cost $2,000 and up.

You don't need automation in a typewriter, anyway, until your practice is very busy. Till then, you can get a very good new machine—the kind that speeds corrections, usually providing two ribbons (one a correction ribbon, the other standard)—such as the I.B.M. Correcting Selectric, my choice, or the less-costly Adler 21-D, Facit, or Royal. Or you can get a reconditioned I.B.M. office model. Don't settle for less, though, than a solidly built office model—electric, to be sure. Yes, I know you can buy a reconditioned manual typewriter for much less. money. But an electric model is much faster and easier to use and—most important—it'll give you a public image money can't buy.

Selecting from all that equipment is one matter; paying for it is another. Don't assume that you'll buy it all out of pocket or float a bank loan. Buying outright is just one of your options—and not necessarily the better of the two basic options open to you. The second option is leasing.

Think of prices in terms of monthly leasing payments, rather than outright purchase. You use business-office equipment month after month, so it's not foolish to pay for it month after month, especially when you can pay lots of small amounts that way, rather than a lump sum. You can buy $5,000 worth of assorted office equipment for about $150 a month or $10,000 worth for about $290 a month.

Maybe you'd be better off going on the hook for that kind of obligation than buying everything on the cheap. So don't be too quick to reject that Correcting Selectric.

There are two basic kinds of leases—operating and financial. The first kind can be defined as any kind that isn't the second, and the second kind is viewed by the Internal Revenue Service as a tax dodge or a probable tax dodge. Basically, it *is* a tax dodge.

To understand the tax reason for leasing, you first have to understand the penalty built into an outright purchase of office equipment or any other kind of capital equipment. To buy a dollar's worth of equipment, you must earn something like two full dollars, so that you can pay a dollar to Uncle Sam in taxes and have the other dollar left for buying the equipment. No one ever really buys, say, an $810 typewriter; the full outlay is $1,620. True, you depreciate—tax-deduct, over a period of years—the full $810 purchase price. But forget about the other $810 that goes to taxes.

The way out is called leasing, if you can get away with it. The I.R.S. likes to think all finance leases are disguised purchases, but that's not true. Business-office equipment, like clinical equipment, does become obsolete, and it does wear out. So there's much to be said for obtaining various kinds of equipment through a finance lease for three years or five years (those are the usual terms) and deciding at the end of the term whether to make the balloon payment at the end and keep the stuff or to trade it in for a newer, better model.

Financially, the big difference to you between buying and leasing is that, as long as the I.R.S. agrees that your lease *is* a lease and not a disguised purchase, you pay $810 for the typewriter and nothing at all to the tax man, and you still tax-deduct the price of the typewriter.

But don't you pay the leasing company for the privilege of leasing? Of course, you do—just as you pay a bank for the privilege of borrowing its money. The leasing fee you pay isn't called interest, but it might as well be; from your point of view, it's the same thing. And leasing companies, like banks, charge different fees for the use of their money. Leasing firms tend to charge more than banks, but some don't charge you very much more.

So, economically, leasing often makes sense. That's not a matter of opinion; it's undeniable fact. "Is buying cheaper or better than leasing?" is the wrong question. You've got to compare a specific purchase deal with a specific lease deal. A good deal on a lease may be as good as or better than a bad deal on a purchase.

The best way to make a finance lease stand up under I.R.S. scrutiny is, first, to deal with a well-established finance leasing firm that knows the tax angles cold and, second, to make sure that the balloon payment at the end is substantial—an amount equal to 10 or 15 per cent of the equipment's purchase price.

You can find such firms in the Yellow Pages for the city where you'll be in practice or in the biggest city nearby. More difficult than finding a leasing company that handles equipment leases for small offices is finding one that will deal with new doctors.

"Look," you'll hear, "I'd like to help you, but you're new in business; you've got no track record. I'd ask you to make out a financial statement, but all the figures would be on the liability side of the page. You've got no assets. Why don't you come back in a couple of years?"

Don't be discouraged when you hear that nonsense; leasing companies come and go, and there are always some around that are eager for business—new-doctor business included.

Is it worth the struggle and the search? That depends not so much on the tax and interest considerations as on your plan, if any, for bringing another doctor into the practice. In a growing practice with new doctors coming in, I strongly prefer leased equipment over purchased equipment. With the lease, the equipment is paid for as it's used. And it's paid for by the practice, rather than by you as an individual investor. If you buy equipment outright, you suffer the tax penalty we just discussed, even if the new doctor pays you for half the nondepreciated value of the equipment. What's more, he pays a tax penalty approximately equal to the amount he pays you. And on top of all that, you, faced with what the I.R.S. calls recapture, may have to give up part of your depreciation deduction. It's easier and often cheaper to lease and let the new doctor come in without any question of his buying into capital equipment.

The question of bringing in another doctor is a whole other matter. Let's take up that subject in the next chapter. But first let me add a happy postscript to my opening crystal-ball-gazing.

I didn't invent that stuff about computers; I'm on safe ground. More than 200 physicians in Pennsylvania, Ohio, Michigan, Indiana, and Florida are, as I write these words, already on real-time, on-line access to a central computer service sold by Medical Data Systems Corp., which provides instant filing and instant access to patients' charts. The terminal gives both visual access and paper copy through a printer. In addition to handling charts, the system provides billing and collection service, insurance-form preparation, surgical scheduling, and instant written communication with other medical offices on the system. It also computes, in a group practice, each doctor's fees and payments—the data needed for a fair, sophisticated compensation system. And it grants access to such information only to those who have been given appropriate security clearance and access coding. The system also does all the office bookkeeping, and it can provide, to any client who's interested, computerized tax returns, payroll preparation, inventory record keeping, and appointment scheduling.

The monthly fee for this service depends on the size of the practice, but it's about $675 for a two-man practice—$157 a week or about $3.92 an hour.

I don't say that you can afford it yet. But in a year or two or three, you may not be able to afford to be without such service. By then, it may be everywhere—but more sophisticated, and perhaps at even less cost.

There *is* a computer in your future.

# 20

## When and how to bring in another doctor

All too often, an established physician brings in a new doctor for the wrong reason or before he's ready to do so. One commonplace reason is that the established doctor wants more time off—but the same income. You can get paid in time or in money; it's awfully hard to get paid in both.

Never mind whether getting both is possible. Just don't take another doctor into your practice expecting to get more time off without giving a little on the income. No matter how many doctors are in a practice, any one doctor's income must depend on his own productivity, the dollars that he himself brings in—unless he makes a living out of the other doctors' pockets. A certain amount of income justifiably flows from a new doctor to his established colleague, but a fair limit is quickly reached.

The desire for companionship is another bad reason to bring in another doctor, understandable as that motivation is. Be sure there's enough work and enough income for both physicians.

## Getting started in private practice

A third bad reason, not nearly as commonplace as those first two but common enough, is a desire to build an empire or a fiefdom. A lord-of-the-manor type, as opposed to a doctor who simply wants to build a big group practice for the good of the community and the doctors involved, jealously protects his practice, his baby, *his* asset—and he treats a new doctor accordingly, giving him little voice in the operation of the practice and a lot less compensation than he deserves.

What are the right reasons for bringing in a new doctor? Your community needs another doctor, and you want to practice with him on fair terms, which I define as terms you could live with if you were the new doctor.

The best way to recruit your new associate is by letting doctor-friends in your community and in other parts of the country know that you've got a good opportunity for a capable doctor and that you're on the lookout. You probably know some of the key people where you trained, so be sure to include them on your list of contacts. Add the names of the executive directors of your county and state medical societies or their placement offices if they've got them, and send a letter to the American Medical Association's placement office in Chicago. You might also try advertising in the publications you regularly see that carry classified advertising— your county medical society bulletin; state medical society journal; and state, regional, and national specialty society journals.

Since you've never had the experience of taking a new doctor into your practice, you run a high risk of settling on the wrong person if your recruiting efforts yield only two or three likely applicants. So in your ad ask each applicant to write you a letter, detailing his training and experience in patient care, and give your own name and address; don't use a blind ad. Be sure to acknowledge each letter immediately on its arrival with a brief, freshly typed letter. It need say no more than something like this:

"I appreciate your replying to my ad in The Journal of the American Medical Association. I've received a number of other replies, and I expect to be receiving still more in the next week or two. When the flow subsides, I'll give all the letters careful review and get back to you. I very much appreciate your interest."

**250**

On the basis of what you receive in the mail, you should have little trouble in identifying one or more potential partners. Get these doctors on the phone. Any questions raised in the letters can be discussed then, and you can ask for references if they weren't supplied in the letters. Ask for the names, addresses, and phone numbers of faculty advisers, chiefs of service, hospital administra-

*(Continued on page 255)*

FIGURE 20-1 ═══════════════════════════════════════

## A Monthly Management Report

As you go along, keep track of production and adjustment figures, as well as charges and professional receipts, striking your totals for those categories daily and monthly. Then you'll have most of the basic data needed for this management system. In addition, you'll need to keep a monthly tally of nonphysician payroll and outlay for office space (rent, utilities, cleaning, etc.). With the information in hand, you can complete this report in about 15 minutes with the help of an electronic calculator. It will give you a reasonable idea of where you're headed and how much you can afford to spend in two key areas of your budget.

### Forecasting Production, Adjustments, and Charges

| | | Example figures | Your figures | Line |
|---|---|---|---|---|
| A. | Production (dollar value of services rendered, without discounting for professional courtesy, poverty, or other consideration) for past 12 months | $166,100 | _____ | A |
| B. | Production for the 12 months preceding that period | $159,700 | _____ | B |
| C. | Gain (+) or loss (−): Line A minus Line B | +$6,400 | _____ | C |
| D. | Percentage gain (+) or loss (−): Line C divided by Line B | +4.008% | _____% | D |
| E. | Production for the past six months | $83,850 | _____ | E |
| F. | Monthly average: Line E divided by 6 | $13,975 | _____ | F |
| G. | Production for the 12 months preceding that period | $162,894 | _____ | G |
| H. | Monthly average: Line G divided by 12 | $13,575 | _____ | H |

# Getting started in private practice

|  |  | Example figures | Your figures | Line |
|---|---|---|---|---|
| I. | Gain (+) or loss (−): Line F minus Line H | +$400 | _____ | I |
| J. | Percentage gain (+) or loss (−): Line I divided by Line H | +2.947% | _____% | J |
| K. | Average production for the past six months: Repeat Line F here | $13,975 | _____ | K |
| L. | Production for the same six months one year previous | $80,400 | _____ | L |
| M. | Monthly average for that period: Line L divided by 6 | $13,400 | _____ | M |
| N. | Gain (+) or loss (−): Line K minus Line M | +$575 | _____ | N |
| O. | Percentage gain (+) or loss (−): Line N divided by Line M | +4.291% | _____% | O |
| P. | Total of Lines D, J, and O | +11.246% | _____% | P |
| Q. | Current rate of growth: Line P divided by 3 | +3.749% | _____% | Q |
| R. | Projected gain (+) or loss (−) in production for the next 12 months: Line Q multiplied by Line A | +$6,227 | _____ | R |
| S. | Now a highly subjective factor: Add or subtract any gain or loss that can reasonably be anticipated due to retirement or recruitment of a doctor, physician's assistant, nurse-practitioner, therapist, or other fee-for-service professional or paraprofessional; move to new office; addition or loss of fee-producing lab, X-ray, or other equipment; and/or other factor: | 0 | _____ | S |
| T. | Production projection: Total Lines A, R, and S | $172,327 | _____ | T |
| U. | Adjustments for the past 12 months | $9,965 | _____ | U |
| V. | Charges for the past 12 months: Line A minus Line U | $156,135 | _____ | V |
| W. | Adjustments as a percentage of production in the past 12 months: Line U divided by Line A | 5.999% | _____ | W |
| X. | Adjustment projection: Line W multiplied by Line T | $10,338 | _____ | X |

| | | Example figures | Your figures | Line |
|---|---|---|---|---|
| **Y.** | Charges projection: Line T minus Line X | $161,989 | _____ | Y |
| **Z.** | Projected charges as a percentage of projected production: Line Y divided by Line T | 94.001% | _____% | ⌐ |

**Forecasting Collection Ratio (C/R) and Receipts**

| | | Example figures | Your figures | Line |
|---|---|---|---|---|
| **AA.** | Charges for the past six months | $81,456 | _____ | AA |
| **BB.** | Professional receipts (payments) for the past six months | $79,419 | _____ | BB |
| **CC.** | Charges for the 12 months preceding that period | $153,814 | _____ | CC |
| **DD.** | Professional receipts for that same period as Line CC | $148,430 | _____ | DD |
| **EE.** | Charges for the past 12 months: Repeat Line V | $156,135 | _____ | EE |
| **FF.** | Professional receipts for that same period as Line EE | $153,480 | _____ | FF |
| **GG.** | C/R Factor 1: Current C/R: Line FF divided by Line EE | 98.300% | _____% | GG |
| **HH.** | C/R Factor 2: Line DD divided by Line CC | 96.500% | _____% | HH |
| **II.** | C/R Factor 3: Line BB divided by Line AA | 97.499% | _____% | II |
| **JJ.** | C/R Factor 4: Add Lines GG, HH, and II | 292.299% | _____% | JJ |
| **KK.** | Collection ratio projection for the next 12 months: Line JJ divided by 3 | 97.433% | _____% | KK |
| **LL.** | Professional receipts projection: Line KK multiplied by Line Y | $157,831 | _____ | LL |

**Budgeting Guidelines**

| | | Example figures | Your figures | Line |
|---|---|---|---|---|
| **MM.** | Your practice's gross payroll, excluding all physicians, for the past 12 months | $24,184 | _____ | MM |
| **NN.** | Payroll factor: Line MM divided by Line A | 14.560% | _____% | NN |
| **OO.** | Payroll budget guideline for next 12 months: Line NN multiplied by Line T | $25,091 | _____ | OO |

| | | Example figures | Your figures | Line |
|---|---|---|---|---|
| **PP.** | Our subjective guideline for the total outlay for equipment payments (rental, leasing payments, loan repayments) and office space (rent, utilities, whatever): Line T multiplied by .095 | $16,371 | _____ | **PP** |

### Summary of Projections and Guidelines

| | | Example figures | Your figures | Line |
|---|---|---|---|---|
| **QQ:** | | | | **QQ:** |
| | **a.** Production (Line T) | $172,327 | _____ | **a** |
| | **b.** Adjustments (Line X) | $10,338 | _____ | **b** |
| | **c.** Charges (Line Y) | $161,989 | _____ | **c** |
| | **d.** Collection ratio (Line KK) | 97.433% | _____% | **d** |
| | **e.** Professional receipts (Line LL) | $157,831 | _____ | **e** |
| | **f.** Payroll (Line OO) | $25,091 | _____ | **f** |
| | **g.** Office space/equipment (Line PP) | $16,371 | _____ | **g** |

### Current Spending Reviewed

| | | Example figures | Your figures | Line |
|---|---|---|---|---|
| **RR.** | Payroll last payday, excluding all physicians | $1,965 | _____ | **RR** |
| **SS.** | Payroll annualized: Line RR multiplied by the number of your paydays yearly: □52 □26 □24 □12 □ _____ | $23,580 | _____ | **SS** |
| **TT.** | Difference between payroll guidelines and your current payroll: Line QQ(f) minus Line SS=Available funds (or expenditure above budgeting guideline) | $1,511 | _____ | **TT** |
| **UU.** | Outlay last month for office space [$ _____] and payments for equipment [$ _____] | $1,625 | _____ | **UU** |
| **VV.** | Space and equipment annualized: Line UU multiplied by 12 | $19,500 | _____ | **VV** |
| **WW.** | Difference between space/equipment guideline and current outlay: Line QQ(g) minus Line VV=Available funds (or expenditure above budgeting guideline) | ($3,129) | _____ | **WW** |

### Notes and Suggestions

_____

tors, chief residents—anyone who is in a position to know the applicants and the quality of their work.

One of the nice things about checking out physicians with the people who train and supervise them is that they tend to pull no punches. It's as if there were some vast agreement that anyone in such a position of authority will take no chance of discrediting his position by giving anything less than an honest appraisal. I say that because on numerous occasions I've been in the company of hospital administrators and chiefs of service when they received referral phone calls, and I've heard their end of the conversation. Someone ought to make tape-recordings of a dozen or so of those conversations and play them back to medical students. The experience would be sobering.

So it's well worth your while to get on the phone, spend a few bucks on long-distance calls, and check out the best of your candidates. Just as quickly as you can, narrow your selection down

*(Continued on page 259)*

FIGURE 20-2 ════════════════════════════════════════

### Are You Ready to Take In a Second Doctor?

| | Example | Your answer | Line |
|---|---|---|---|
| **A.** Most doctors who practice comfortably and successfully in nonsolo practice seem to be better organized than average, enjoy private practice, are not especially competitive, are considered good managers and bosses, delegate easily and well, and run offices with happy atmospheres. Does that sound like you? | ☒ Yes ☐ No | ☐ Yes ☐ No | **A** |
| **B.** Would your employees accept a second doctor happily? | ☒ Yes ☐ No | ☐ Yes ☐ No | **B** |
| **C.** If it turns out that one or more of your assistants gives the newcomer significant aggravation (whether from some false sense of loyalty to you or a personality clash), are you prepared to discipline and, if necessary, fire? | ☒ Yes ☐ No | ☐ Yes ☐ No | **C** |

# Getting started in private practice

| | Example | Your answer | Line |
|---|---|---|---|
| **D.** If your wife now works in the office, will she get out once the new doctor arrives? | ☒ Yes ☐ No | ☐ Yes ☐ No | **D** |
| **E.** If you can't give a Yes answer to this question, you can forget about the rest of this worksheet and about taking another doctor into your office. On balance, do the subjective factors support your taking in another doctor? | ☒ Yes ☐ No | ☐ Yes ☐ No | **E** |

## Need for Another Doctor

| | Example | Your answer | Line |
|---|---|---|---|
| **F.** What's the resident civilian population of the community you serve? You can get the figure from your Chamber of Commerce or County Planning Board | 47,500 | —— | **F** |
| **G.** How many doctors in the community are now practicing your specialty? Your county medical society probably has a count | 16 | —— | **G** |
| **H.** Population per doctor: Line F divided by Line G | 2,969 | —— | **H** |
| **I.** Figure 20-3 shows the estimated population range required to support a doctor. For your speciality, what's the minimum figure shown? | 2,700 | —— | **I** |
| **J.** What are other doctors in the area doing? Retiring? Cutting back? Bringing in partners of their own? On balance, does the competitive situation indicate that you're probably safe in bringing in another doctor? | ☒ Yes ☐ No | ☐ Yes ☐ No | **J** |
| **K.** What about informed outsiders like the hospital administrator and the county medical society's executive director: Do they seem to agree that another doctor is needed? | ☒ Yes ☐ No | ☐ Yes ☐ No | **K** |
| **L.** Considering the evidence, do you see a need for another doctor of your specialty in the community? If No, reconsider bringing in a second doctor now. | ☒ Yes ☐ No | ☐ Yes ☐ No | **L** |

## Suitability of Your Office

**M.** Highly productive practices have ample examining rooms available for each doctor seeing patients at any given time—often four or more rooms, depending on specialty, but in any

|  | Example | Your answer | Line |
|---|---|---|---|
| case enough per doctor so there's no wasted time between patients. Do you have even enough rooms to meet your own needs? | ☒ Yes<br>☐ No | ☐ Yes<br>☐ No | **M** |
| **N.** Would you and your partner be seeing patients in the office at the same time? If Yes, are there enough rooms to keep both of you fully productive? | ☐ Yes<br>☒ No | ☐ Yes<br>☐ No | **N** |
| **O.** If you replied No at Line N, are you prepared to build a new office building or move into a bigger office reasonably soon after the second doctor's arrival? | ☒ Yes<br>☐ No | ☐ Yes<br>☐ No | **O** |
| **P.** On balance, will the office-space situation deter bringing in a second doctor? | ☐ Yes<br>☒ No | ☐ Yes<br>☐ No | **P** |

## Some Final Considerations

|  | Example | Your answer | Line |
|---|---|---|---|
| **Q.** Perhaps you don't need another doctor as much as you need more paramedical assistants, such as a physician's assistant, nurse-practitioner, midwife, physical therapist, or audiologist. Do you need to give that more consideration before recruiting a doctor? | ☐ Yes<br>☒ No | ☐ Yes<br>☐ No | **Q** |
| **R.** Do you and the community need another doctor as much as you need more time off? If time off is your real motivation, have you considered that you'll carry the burden of a two-man practice when covering your partner's time off and that respite may not come until you've added a third doctor? Have you considered a better coverage arrangement as the alternative to bringing in a second doctor? | ☒ Yes<br>☐ No | ☐ Yes<br>☐ No | **R** |
| **S.** How possessive do you feel about your patients and your practice? Are you willing to work with another doctor as a full and equal partner? | ☒ Yes<br>☐ No | ☐ Yes<br>☐ No | **S** |
| **T.** Are you prepared to offer attractive terms? | ☒ Yes<br>☐ No | ☐ Yes<br>☐ No | **T** |

## The Decision

|  | Example | Your answer | Line |
|---|---|---|---|
| **U.** Are you ready to take in another doctor? | ☒ Yes<br>☐ No | ☐ Yes<br>☐ No | **U** |

FIGURE 20-3 ═══════════════════════════════════════════

## How Much Population
## to Support One Doctor?

The estimates vary, sometimes widely. Henry Wechsler, Ph.D., published some estimates in his Handbook of Medical Specialties, published in 1976 by Human Sciences Press, New York. I've rounded off his figures and added my own column on the apparent need for more (+) or fewer (−) persons in the various specialties. In obstetrics and gynecology, for instance, the patient-doctor ratio indicates a slight shortage of doctors; in my opinion, there's not really much need for more physicians in this specialty.

| Need | Specialty | Actual population per doctor | Estimated population needed per doctor |
|---|---|---|---|
| + | Allergy and immunology | 117,243 | n.a. |
|  | Anesthesiology | 19,182 | 17,500-38,500 |
| + | Colon and rectal surgery | 334,478 | n.a. |
| + | Dermatology | 55,251 | 43,500-45,500 |
| + | Family and general practice | 4,197 | 2,300-4,000 |
| − | General surgery | 7,632 | 8,400-11,600 |
| + | Internal medicine | 5,083 | 2,700-3,600 |
|  | Internal medicine subspecialties | 27,593 | n.a. |
| − | Neurological surgery | 83,290 | 90,900-100,000 |
| − | Neurology | 77,206 | 77,000-100,000 |
|  | Obstetrics and gynecology | 11,240 | 10,200-11,000 |
| − | Ophthalmology | 21,520 | 20,800-40,000 |
| − | Orthopedic surgery | 21,559 | 23,800-27,800 |
| + | Otolaryngology | 43,000 | 30,300-43,500 |
|  | Pathology | 25,441 | 22,700-76,900 |
| + | Pediatrics | 11,925 | 6,600-7,100 |
| + | Physical medicine and rehabilitation | 180,830 | 100,000 |
|  | Plastic surgery | 110,908 | 66,700-500,000 |
|  | Preventive medicine specialties | 86,671 | n.a. |
| − | Psychiatry | 10,422 | 10,000-62,500 |
| − | Radiology | 15,863 | 17,900-32,300 |
| + | Thoracic surgery | 127,267 | n.a. |
|  | Urology | 36,240 | 29,400-55,600 |

to the one, two, or three candidates worth the investment of a little traveling money. Invite each candidate and his spouse to come visit—to spend a couple of days with you, to look over the office and the community, to talk. You needn't make it a blank-check invitation; you can tell a candidate that you'll be happy to give him a check for $200, or whatever, "to help pay your expenses." Make the figure large enough to cover travel, lodging, and meals. You can always be lavish later, if you're so inclined, when you pay the moving expenses of the candidate who's to join you.

Once you're convinced that you've found the right person—someone who can pull his own weight, develop a strong patient following of his own, do a good job with his patients and yours—offer him good terms. As far as I'm concerned, the best possible deal a young doctor can get is an arrangement that will let him do as well clinically and financially in a multidoctor practice as he could do in solo practice. In fact, he should do even better.

Remember: Every income-sharing arrangement is automatically an expense-sharing arrangement, too. And though another doctor does mean an accompanying increase in certain expenditures—supplies consumed, a part-time nurse, possibly a larger office—it's also true that some of the expenses now borne by you alone will be shared, giving you a financial gain. A dollar saved in overhead is, after all, a dollar more of income. So you stand to gain financially every time you add a doctor to the practice, even if he doesn't pay you a dime for the privilege.

That's not to say, though, that you're not entitled to a little something extra. Your administrative ability has established a growing practice, you've assembled equipment and office space, you've acquired a patient following, you've trained a staff in the systems and procedures that make your professional life bearable and financially rewarding, and you'll oversee things while the new doctor settles in.

By and large, it takes three or four years for a new doctor in practice to develop something approaching his full abilities. That's why many of your older colleagues have used that time as the period leading to full partnership. That term properly means a full

*(Continued on page 266)*

FIGURE 20-4 ═══════════════════════════════════════════

## Points to Cover
## When Bringing In Another Doctor

**A.** Capital to be contributed by each doctor:
Dr. _____ $_____
Dr. _____ $_____

Total:  $30,000   _____ **A**

**B.** Method of compensation:
- ☐ Tenure: After one year of straight salary for the newcomer, 30% of net practice income in Year 2, 40% in Year 3, 50% in Year 4 and thereafter; the balance to the senior doctor

- ☐ Tenure: As detailed in Schedule A (attach)

- ☐ Production: Net practice income to be shared in same ratio as production (production defined as full value of services rendered before adjustment for courtesy and poverty)

- ☐ Production: Net practice income to be shared in same ratio as charges (charges defined as value of services rendered after adjustment for courtesy and poverty)

- ☐ Production: Net practice income to be shared in same ratio as receipts (payments to each doctor for services rendered)

- ☐ Production: Basic overhead of the practice to be shared equally and charged against each doctor's receipts (basic overhead defined as office rents, utilities, and all other deductible business expenses not treated as chargebacks to a doctor's compensation fund)

- ☐ Production: Basic overhead to be shared in same ratio as production and charged against each doctor's receipts

- ☐ Production: As detailed in Schedule B (attach)   DONE   ☐ **B**

**C.** Time off per year for combined vacation, convention, and sick days:
- ☐ As each doctor elects, subject to agreement by second doctor on working schedule and coverage
- ☐ Dr. _____ : Year 1 _____, Year 2 _____, Year 3 _____, Year 4 _____, Year 5 _____

Dr. _____ : Year 1 ____, Year 2 ____,
Year 3 ____, Year 4 ____, Year 5 ____     DONE     ☐   **C**

**D.** Determine newcomer's guaranty for first year:
- ☐ None
- ☐ $ _____ salary plus the following:
  - ☐ Malpractice insurance premium
  - ☐ $ _____ of term life insurance premium
  - ☐ $ _____ for health-expense
    reimbursement, including premiums for
    health and disability insurance protection
  - ☐ $ _____ as reimbursement for
    professional car expenses
  - ☐ $ _____ as reimbursement for meetings,
    seminars, continuing education expenses
  - ☐ $ _____ for the following: _____
    _____
- ☐ $ _____ compensation fund; doctor to
  determine its distribution for salary, bonus,
  expense reimbursements, employee
  benefits; to ☐ include ☐ exclude the P.C.'s
  payments for payroll taxes directly resulting
  from doctor's employment (including Social
  Security contribution and state and Federal
  unemployment, disability insurance, and
  workmen's compensation taxes)     DONE     ☐   **D**

**E.** Determine newcomer's obligation to pay
an administrative fee to senior doctor for
administrative services provided by the latter:
- ☐ An amount equal to the practice's gross
  practice income for the 36 months preceding
  the month in which the newcomer joins the
  practice [$ _____]; divided by 3 [$ _____];
  multiplied by .25 [$ _____]; said sum to be
  transferred from the newcomer's compensation
  fund to the senior doctor's compensation fund
  in 60 equal monthly installments, at 8%
  interest, determined by multiplying said sum by
  .02028 [$ _____], the first of the 60
  consecutive transfers to take place in the 13th
  month after the newcomer's arrival in the
  practice; without adjustment for any
  administrative labors to be provided by the
  newcomer, if any; such labors to be determined
  from time to time as the parties agree.
- ☐ As detailed in Schedule C (attach)     DONE     ☐   **E**

**F.** Determine purchase of doctor's shareholdings in
the P.C. in the event of death:
- ☐ Surviving partner to have first option to
purchase the shares for book value; treasury to
have second option; another incoming doctor
to have third option

- ☐ As detailed in Schedule D (attach)  DONE  ☐ **F**

**G.** Determine purchase of doctor's shareholdings in
the P.C. in the event of total disability:
- ☐ Surviving partner to have first option to
purchase the shares for book value; treasury to
have second option; another incoming doctor
to have third option; total disability determined
by payment of first disability-insurance benefit
by the carrier of a policy with an exclusion
period of ☐ 6 months ☐ 12 months; options to
be opened on receipt of said payment.

- ☐ As detailed in Schedule E (attach)  DONE  ☐ **G**

**H.** Determine purchase of doctor's shareholdings in
the P.C. in the event of his resignation, whether for
retirement or other reason, after becoming a full
and equal shareholder:
- ☐ As detailed in Line F

- ☐ As detailed in Schedule F (attach)  DONE  ☐ **H**

**I.** Determine purchase of a doctor's shareholdings in
the event of his termination for cause; cause
defined as conviction of a felony in any state, loss
of license to practice medicine or surgery in any
state, or loss of hospital privileges through
disciplinary proceedings at any hospital:
- ☐ As in Line F

- ☐ As detailed in Schedule G (attach)  DONE  ☐ **I**

**J.** Determine disposition of doctor's accounts
receivable in the event of his death:
- ☐ If compensation is based on production (Line
B), normal distribution to continue for a period
of ☐ 12 months ☐ _____ months from the date
of death

- ☐ As detailed in Schedule H (attach)  DONE  ☐ **J**

**K.** Determine disposition of doctor's accounts
receivable in the event of his total disability:
☐ As in Line F; total disability as determined
in Line G

☐ As detailed in Schedule I (attach)       DONE       ☐ **K**

**L.** Determine disposition of doctor's accounts
receivable in event of his resignation after attaining
shareholdings equal to those of senior doctor:
☐ If compensation is based on production (Line
B), normal distribution to continue for a period
of ☐ 12 months ☐ _____ months from date of
resignation

☐ As detailed in Schedule J (attach)       DONE       ☐ **L**

**M.** Determine disposition of doctor's accounts
receivable in event of his resignation before
attaining shareholdings equal to those of the senior
doctor:
☐ No distribution after date of resignation

☐ As detailed in Schedule K (attach)       DONE       ☐ **M**

**N.** Determine disposition of doctor's accounts
receivable in event of his termination by P.C.:
☐ If a full and equal shareholder, as in Line H

☐ If less than a full and equal shareholder, as in
Line L, unless termination is for cause; cause
defined as conviction of a felony in any state,
loss of license to practice medicine through
disciplinary proceedings in any state, loss of
hospital privileges through disciplinary
proceedings at any hospital

☐ If terminated for cause before becoming a full
and equal shareholder, as in Line M

☐ As detailed in Schedule L (attach)       DONE       ☐ **N**

**O.** Determine the protection of the newcomer in the
event of termination for less than cause:
☐ Accounts receivable distribution as in Line M
plus termination allowance equal to: Total of
W-2 compensation paid from first day in the
practice [$_____] multiplied by .166
[$_____] or $2,500, whichever is greater

☐ As detailed in Schedule M (attach)       DONE       ☐ **O**

**P.** Determine the protection of the senior doctor in the event of the resignation of the newcomer in order to enter into competition:
- ☐ If the newcomer is less than a full and equal partner, distribution of accounts receivable as in Line M; payment by the newcomer to the senior doctor as a fee for introduction into the professional community in the same amount as in Line O
- ☐ As detailed in Schedule N (attach)    DONE    ☐ **P**

**Q.** Determine what's to happen in the event of an agreement of full and equal shareholders to part company for reasons other than death, total disability, voluntary resignation for retirement or other purposes, or termination for cause:
- ☐ Doctor with greatest tenure to exercise first option on continued occupancy of office, including any satellite offices; office phone numbers to be changed; accounts receivable to be distributed as in Line J, all employees to be offered option of continued employment with either doctor without change in compensation for period of three months; name of the corporation to be changed to any other name approved by doctor with greatest tenure; each doctor to give an announcement to whomever he wishes, wording to be approved in writing in advance of distribution by each and every doctor with full and equal shareholdings
- ☐ As detailed in Schedule O (attach)    DONE    ☐ **Q**

**R.** Determine the manner in which any disputes are to be settled:
- ☐ Through binding arbitration conducted under the rules of the American Arbitration Association, New York
- ☐ As detailed in Schedule P (attach)    DONE    ☐ **R**

**S.** The present name of the practice, its principal office address, its published phone number(s):

_____

_____

_____ ZIP: _____

Phone(s): _____    DONE    ☐ **S**

**T.** Tax details of the practice at present:
☐ Proprietorship ☐ Partnership
☐ Professional corporation ☐ Other: _____

Employer identification number: _____

Fiscal year ends: _____

Federal tax form last filed: ☐ Schedule C, Form 1040 ☐ Form 1065 ☐ Form 1120 ☐ Form 1120S ☐ _____

Retirement plan in effect: ☐ Keogh ☐ P.C. profit-sharing ☐ P.C. pension plan ☐ Both P.C. profit-sharing and P.C. pension plan
☐ _____

Retirement-plan designer (name, address):

_____

_____

_____ ZIP: _____
Retirement-plan administrator if different from the above: _____

_____

_____ ZIP: _____
Accountant: _____

_____

_____ ZIP: _____

DONE    ☐    **T**

**U.** Identification of doctors in the practice, including newcomer(s):

| Name of doctor | Date of birth | Soc. Sec.# | State medical lic. # | M.D. D.O.? | Home address |
|---|---|---|---|---|---|
| | | | | | |
| | | | | | |

**V.** Date newcomer joined or will join the practice: _____

**W.** Additional comment:

The above indicates our agreement:
Signed:

_____    Date: _____

_____    Date: _____

and equal say in policy and practice administration, but it doesn't necessarily mean full ownership of the practice assets.

Take real estate. Your practice needs the use of office space, but that's not the same as saying that your practice ought to *own* it. A landlord can just as easily own it, and the identity of the landlord has nothing to do with the ongoing administration of the practice, as long as his terms are fair. If the landlord is you, offering a part ownership of the property to the new doctor is strictly a question of investment, not an appropriate condition of his joining you. If you're sincere about wanting to bring in an associate, forget about making his investment in your real estate venture a condition of association. Just set the rental to the practice—to your professional corporation—at a fair level, one that's consistent with your community's going rate for similar office space.

What about payment for the other assets—the equipment, leasehold improvements, fixtures and furnishings, cash advanced, supplies on hand, goodwill? A direct investment is unnecessary. The value of such assets can be tallied and paid for indirectly out of funds generated by the new doctor's production. That's nothing more than a play on the old 30-40-50 per cent income-sharing arrangement used for generations by your older colleagues, except that their way was all hit-or-miss, with no systematic effort to

FIGURE 20-5 ═══════════════════════════════════════

### Keeping Score With a Partner

How can you keep score when you bring in another doctor? It's not so hard if your assistant identifies the doctor who provides the services to a patient—as here, by an initial in the provider column on the left. At day's end she runs a total on each doctor and adds that adding-machine tape to the two others attached to the daysheet. The daily totals and later the monthly totals can go on individual tally sheets like those shown in Chapter 9. Keeping score, too, on adjustments, charges, and payments for each doctor is a little more work, but it's not hard to do. Just carry the doctor's initial through to the patient's ledger card. Later, when a payment arrives, an assistant posts it on the ledger card and at that time can note which doctor is to receive credit. A partial payment goes to the oldest debt.

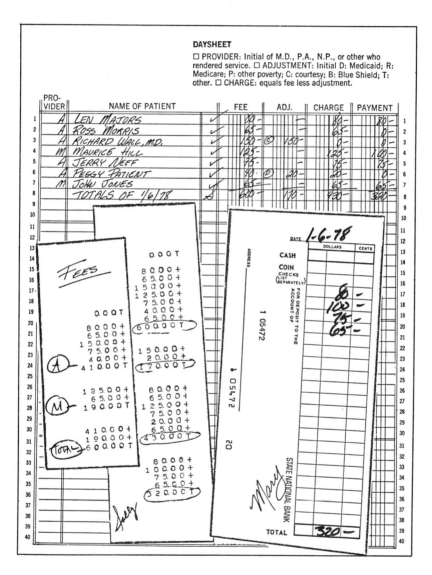

**DAYSHEET**

☐ PROVIDER: Initial of M.D., P.A., N.P., or other who rendered service. ☐ ADJUSTMENT: Initial D: Medicaid; R: Medicare; P: other poverty; C: courtesy; B: Blue Shield; T: other. ☐ CHARGE: equals fee less adjustment.

| PRO-VIDER | NAME OF PATIENT | | FEE | ADJ. | CHARGE | PAYMENT |
|---|---|---|---|---|---|---|
| A | LEN MAJORS | ✓ | 80 - | - | 80 - | 80 - |
| A | ROSS MORRIS | ✓ | 65 - | - | 65 - | 0 - |
| A | RICHARD WALL, M.D. | ✓ | 150 - | Ⓒ 150 - | 0 - | 0 - |
| M | MAURICE HILL | ✓ | 125 - | - | 125 - | 100 - |
| A | JERRY NEFF | ✓ | 75 - | - | 75 - | 75 - |
| A | PEGGY PATIENT | ✓ | 40 - | Ⓒ 20 - | 20 - | 0 - |
| M | JOHN JONES | ✓ | 65 - | - | 65 - | 65 - |
| | TOTALS OF 1/6/78 | | 600 - | 170 - | 430 - | 320 - |

FEES

```
                    0 0 0 T
              8 0.0 0 +
              6 5.0 0 +
            1 5 0.0 0 +
            1 2 5.0 0 +
              7 5.0 0 +
              4 0.0 0 +
              6 5.0 0 +
         0 0 0 T      6 0 0.0 0 T
    8 0.0 0 +
    6 5.0 0 +
  1 5 0.0 0 +       1 5 0.0 0 +
    7 5.0 0 +         2 0.0 0 +
    4 0.0 0 T      1 7 0.0 0 T
Ⓐ 4 1 0.0 0 T

    1 2 5.0 0 +    8 0.0 0 +
      6 5.0 0 +    6 5.0 0 +
Ⓜ 1 9 0.0 0 T    1 2 5.0 0 +
                    7 5.0 0 +
                    2 0.0 0 +
    4 1 0.0 0 +    6 5.0 0 +
    1 9 0.0 0 +  4 3 0.0 0 T
TOTAL 6 0 0.0 0 T

                  8 0.0 0 +
                1 0 0.0 0 +
                  7 5.0 0 +
                  6 5.0 0 +
                3 2 0.0 0 T
```

DATE 1-6-78

| | DOLLARS | CENTS |
|---|---|---|
| CASH | | |
| COIN | | |
| CHECKS (LIST SEPARATELY) | | |
| | 80 - | |
| | 100 - | |
| | 75 - | |
| | 65 - | |

ADDRESS

1 05472

↓ 05472

20

FOR DEPOSIT TO THE ACCOUNT OF

Mary

STATE NATIONAL BANK

TOTAL  320 —

determine if the arrangement was fair to either party. My approach provides such a determination on a continuing, monthly basis. The fairest arrangement I know is built into Figure 20-4.

That arrangement divides the office overhead in proportion to each doctor's production and credits incoming payments to the doctor who provided the service. As was discussed in Chapter 5, identifying which doctor provided a service is a simple matter, as is identifying the payment for that service. Just be sure that you keep score on a daily basis. If you do that, it's easy to tot up the daily totals each month, to add up the monthly scores, and to show the totals for the past 12 months. Again, *you* don't have to do it; your financial secretary or anyone else who knows how to use an adding machine can do the work. It's not calculus.

Figure 20-4 also includes an administrative factor, a credit to the senior doctor in 36 equal and consecutive monthly installments as compensation to him for his administrative and other contributions. The amount of compensation is related to the value of the practice, based on the premise that the healthier the practice, the more valuable its administration.

Figure 20-4 eliminates the following from consideration: any ownership of real estate, since it's to be treated as a completely separate investment matter; the need for the new doctor to buy into this investment; and any need for a restrictive covenant.

In the past couple of years, I've counseled against restrictive covenants because many courts of law have held them to be unfair, illegal, and unenforceable. But never mind the legal question; it's also bad management. If the new doctor turns out to be a dud, what do you care if he opens up in the same county or across the street or down the hall? He'll never become serious competition, anyway. On the other hand, why should you risk being exploited by some freeloader who uses you as an entree to the community, lines of referral, and patients? There's nothing wrong with his doing that—as long as you're properly compensated.

The worksheets in this chapter are companions to Figure 5-1 in Chapter 5, the one that discussed the possibility of starting practice with a doctor-friend or two. If you do that, the worksheets in this chapter can be used by the two or three of you from the start.

# 21

# Some final words on family financial security

I began this book by telling you a little about Dr. Bodner, the fellow I was lunching with at that splendid old Southern country club. Well, the reason we were meeting was to discuss the biggest problem in Dr. Bodner's life—and he didn't even know he had a problem. I'd been seeing him every three months for two years, so I'd come to know him pretty well. His wife had died several years before, and now he thought he wanted to close his practice and accept his daughter's invitation to retire to San Diego, where he could be close to her and her family and enjoy that beautiful southern California coast in his declining years. I figured I knew better.

"To begin with, I'm not so sure that you can afford to retire," I told him, "at least not fully. I like your new Mercedes, your country club, that big house you live in, your housekeeper, and your life style, but the fact of the matter is that you don't have much put away, not even when you include the proceeds you'd realize by selling the house. If you try to live off the earnings of your liquid capital, you'll live very, very modestly. If you draw from capital for living expenses, you still won't live as comfortably as you do here and now. No way.

"But more to the point," I continued, "what do you mean *retire?* I've known you long enough to know that you love every minute here in practice. I see it on your face and in your walk, I see it when you talk with patients, and you told me as much yourself.

"Retirement isn't running off to Florida to drown worms in a canal or to southern California to watch the sunset. Oh, it is, if that's what you really want to do. And I can see where that would be a big deal if you worked in some boring factory job or were killing yourself by working on a farm or in a mine or otherwise doing work you hate, but you don't have that problem. Fishing or sunset-watching would bore you stiff. That's not retirement, anyway. Retirement is doing what you love most—and you've been doing it

FIGURE 21-1

## Representative Annual Premiums for $500,000 of Yearly Renewable Term Life Insurance

Prices vary by company and may change within a company from time to time. The premiums for such protection in the company you select may be higher or lower than these figures:

| Age | Premium | Age | Premium | Age | Premium |
|-----|---------|-----|---------|-----|---------|
| 30 | $ 735 | 36 | $ 834 | 46 | $1,728 |
| 31 | 744 | 37 | 873 | 47 | 1,884 |
| 32 | 756 | 38 | 927 | 48 | 2,058 |
| 33 | 765 | 39 | 993 | 49 | 2,253 |
| 34 | 780 | 40 | 1,068 | 50 | 2,466 |
| 35 | 804 | | | | |
| | | 41 | 1,152 | 51 | 2,700 |
| | | 42 | 1,248 | 52 | 2,952 |
| | | 43 | 1,347 | 53 | 3,228 |
| | | 44 | 1,461 | 54 | 3,525 |
| | | 45 | 1,524 | 55 | 3,852 |

all your working life. You've been 'retired' since you were 28!''

In the end, Dr. Bodner, who truly did miss seeing his daughter and her family, took a little more time off, bought a condominium apartment near San Diego (which he rents out 10 months of each year), and is generally to be found in his vacation home when he's not home working. The arrangement suits him fine, but I think a factor contributing at least as much to his health and well-being is that he's happier with his working life than ever before, because he now realizes that he truly did retire when he entered private practice 'way back when. He takes great pride in his competence, his office and the way it functions, his position of eminence in the community, and the high regard in which he's held by patients. "Why would anyone want to leave all that?" he said to me on the phone not long ago.

He's right. Private practice can be hard, heart-breaking work at times, but people do it and stay with it because they love it. Those who do not love it should get out of it and into industry or research or something that they can enjoy.

If you're among the people who love private practice and belong there, you ought to appreciate what you've got right from the start. The appreciation alone ought to make your life more enjoyable. Of the earth's 4,500,000,000 people, how many—1 per cent?—are privileged to be not just gainfully employed but passing each working day doing exactly what gives them fulfillment and pleasure? So protect what you've got and what you'll build in the professional life that lies before you. But put it all in perspective. Be among the few who truly appreciate all that they've got.

The protection part involves three basic considerations— your financial future, your financial present, and your practice management.

• *Your financial future.* Unlike Dr. Bodner, you've got pension and tax laws that offer you a chance for financial security that's almost beyond belief. You've seen the figures, the tables, the projections. You know that a retirement, pension, or profit-sharing plan doesn't really mean retirement in the traditional sense of old age but is really the misleading term applied to the best and most exciting tax-sheltered investment opportunity there is. And you know that your

**271**

own retirement plan will assure your family's financial security.

All the financial projections I've made in this book are at 8 per cent, which is a trifle less than the yield offered by savings institutions' long-term savings certificates. Not all savings institutions offer that much, but so many do that it's safe to assume you can easily find that much of a return for your professional corporation's retirement plan, no matter where you live. Besides, the savings institutions can freely do business across state lines. No matter where you live, your long-term savings account is only a postage stamp away.

You can, if you wish, be more venturesome and go for more than 8 per cent. That's up to you. The historic rate of growth of common stocks listed on the New York Stock Exchange is a smidgen above 9 per cent. You can nail down 8 to 10 per cent interest by buying certain new bond issues or outstanding issues selling at discounts. Or you can invest in bond funds; they're offered by

FIGURE 21-2 ==========================================

### A Sampling of Low-Premium
### Life-Insurance Companies

The secret to life insurance is to buy only term protection in the amount you need and to buy less as you need less. However, most companies try to sell policies with a so-called savings feature, often called whole life or ordinary life insurance. The first-year premium for that kind of insurance can run at least three times as much as for yearly renewable term insurance, which some companies guarantee to be renewable even to age 100.

Among the few companies that specialize in term coverage are these:

☐ Continental Assurance, 310 South Michigan Blvd., Chicago, Ill. 60604; (312) 822-5000
☐ Great Southern Life, 3121 Buffalo Speedway, Houston, Tex. 77006; (713) 622-2000
☐ National Fidelity Life, 1002 Walnut St., Kansas City, Mo. 64106; (816) 842-6120
☐ Old Line Life, 707 North 11th St., Milwaukee, Wis. 53233; (414) 271-2820
☐ Southwestern Life, 1807 Ross Ave., Dallas, Tex. 75201; (214) 742-9101
☐ United Investors Life, 1 Crown Center, Kansas City, Mo. 64108; (816) 283-4242

mutual-fund organizations, stockbrokers, banks, and insurance companies. There are even Government securities that offer 8 to 10 per cent, and you can get the same return by investing in some corporate notes, mortgages, preferred stocks, and common stocks of utilities, among other solidly based companies. For that matter, it's often possible to get a relatively safe 10 to 12 per cent in utility companies' preferred stocks and some utility, financial, and industrial bonds rated A, Aa, and Aaa.

You may even be able to get more than 12 per cent—perhaps as much as 16 per cent—on bonds rated by Moody's at Baa or higher, on convertible bonds, and on the South African gold-mine stocks known as Kaffirs.

I don't mean to tell you how you should invest your retirement-plan money or any other funds. That subject is covered in other books, not this one. My point is simply that it is possible to go for more than the basic 8 per cent on your investment money without going to Las Vegas.

Remember, though: You don't need to acquire the investment sophistication that many people like Dr. Bodner felt they had to rely on. A tax-free yield of 8 per cent in your retirement plan is equal to something like a 16 per cent yield outside the plan, and it's sure easier to get an 8 per cent return on a retirement-plan investment than a 16 per cent return on a personal investment.

That's not to say that personal investments are to be avoided. Some can be more for fun than for money—paintings, prints and photographs, coins and stamps, tennis centers, pet breeding centers and stables, jewelry and precious stones, resort condominiums in San Diego or Spain or anywhere, even farms. In fact, almost any family business can be fun. And who says all your kids must grow up to become doctors or lawyers or brilliant scientists or even graduate from college, for that matter? The one who decides to devote full time to managing the family business can start an investment program through his own retirement plan and build a personal fortune of his own. Today, the business doesn't even have to be a roaring success to make its key employee wealthy.

• *Your financial present.* I once looked down my nose at anyone who tried to be his own expert, especially in such basic financial matters as taxes and insurance. Life is increasingly complex, and it's tough enough to keep up with the technical changes in one's own field, whether medicine or management, without becoming an expert in another. That's a compelling reason to rely on those who make a full-time study of taxes or insurance or investments or any other area of vital interest to you. Every professional who takes his work seriously, like you, works hard at keeping up.

If only it were an easy matter to find the kind of expert assistance you need. You read Chapter 3, so you know I have

FIGURE 21-3 ═══════════════════════════════════════════════

### The Nation's 10 Largest Investment Companies

Big doesn't necessarily mean best, and it sure doesn't necessarily mean best for you. But of the hundreds of investment companies doing business today, these can be considered the measuring posts on such matters as research and other customer services. But, when dealing with any investment company, remember that a stockbroker (also called an account executive and a customer's man, among other titles) is a salesman and earns his money from commissions on your transactions—not from serving as a portfolio manager or investment adviser. However, some of these major firms have investment-management divisions that earn professional fees for advice and portfolio management and not a penny from sales commissions. The addresses shown here are for home offices; check your phone book for local offices.

☐ Merrill Lynch Pierce Fenner & Smith, 1 Liberty Plaza, New York, N.Y. 10016; (212) 766-7416
☐ Salomon Brothers, 1 New York Plaza, New York, N.Y. 10004; (212) 747-7000
☐ Bache Halsey Stuart, 100 Gold St., New York, N.Y. 10038; (212) 791-1000
☐ E. F. Hutton, 1 Battery Park Plaza, New York, N.Y. 10004; (212) 742-5000
☐ Loeb Rhoades, 42 Wall St., New York, N.Y. 10005; (212) 483-6000
☐ Paine Webber Jackson & Curtis Inc., 140 Broadway, New York, N.Y. 10005; (212) 437-2121
☐ Goldman Sachs, 55 Broad St., New York, N.Y. 10004; (212) 676-8000
☐ Dean Witter Reynolds, Inc., 130 Liberty Plaza, New York, N.Y. 10016; (212) 437-3000
☐ Blyth Eastman Dillon & Co., Inc., 1 Chase Manhattan Plaza, New York, N.Y. 10005; (212) 785-9000
☐ First Boston Corporation, 20 Exchange Pl., New York, N.Y. 10005; (212) 344-1515

about the same attitude toward life-insurance salespeople that Paul Revere had toward King George. I feel the same about tax advisers who parrot the I.R.S. line, accountants and lawyers who don't keep up with developments in their fields, and salesmen who masquerade as consultants. Rather than suggest that you swallow hard and take your chances with any of these people, I'd rather advise you to be your own expert.

In taxes, that's not really so hard. All the basic publications that pros rely on are readily available to you, and acquiring them—from such tax publishers as Commerce Clearing House, Prentice-Hall, and Research Institute of America—costs far less than putting a tax expert on retainer. If your spouse has a head for figures and has no career, let him or her consider being your family tax adviser. He or she can study books, keep up with tax journals and newsletters, go to seminars. Brokerage houses and banks are constantly running free and low-cost seminars on taxes and investments. For instance, Merrill Lynch, Pierce, Fenner & Smith, the nation's biggest brokerage firm, ran a free, month-long seminar on the 1976 Tax Reform Act in many of its 220 offices. Many leading banks also ran free or low-priced programs on the big new tax changes.

In fact, tax seminars and workshops abound, and you can find out about many of them from ads in publications that themselves are great sources of information and education to the serious do-it-yourself financial expert. I mean such publications as The New York Times, The Wall Street Journal, and five magazines that are, in my opinion, the best in the country on practical information for consumers: Better Homes and Gardens (which carries an excellent package of articles on personal finances), Changing Times, Consumer Reports, Medical Economics, and Money. You'll find their addresses, along with those of some good financial book clubs and publishers, in Figure 21-6.

The financial companion to investments is insurance. From the earlier chapters of this book, you know that yearly renewable term insurance is your best life insurance buy and that you can buy all you need in a professional-corporation group life-insurance plan that covers you, any other doctors in your practice, and other employees who work 1,000 hours a year or more. How much insurance you buy is important, because, though your financial future lies with tax-sheltered retirement-plan investments, your family's financial security for the present and immediate future probably depends on life insurance. How much coverage you need depends on a number of variables, including your spouse's income-producing ability, but a rough guide is enough coverage to provide income equal to about 80 per cent of current family spending.

Personal liability insurance is the second most important coverage for you. It includes malpractice, office insurance, and, if you can find any, umbrella insurance. Once widely available in amounts of coverage ranging from $1,000,000 to $10,000,000, umbrella insurance has all but disappeared from the market. Ten years ago, you could buy such coverage for relatively little. But personal liability suits resulted in so many big-dollar awards that the companies writing such insurance wished they'd never had the idea; nearly all stopped offering the coverage. So you may find it impossible to blanket your various specific liability coverages with

---

FIGURE 21-4 ═══════════════════════════════════════════

### A Sampling of Leading Disability Insurers

The kind of insurance sold by these disability insurers is more costly than the group disability insurance endorsed by your specialty and state medical societies. But the group plans have a bad history of cancellation. If your group's plan is discontinued, you may need to pass a physical examination to buy replacement coverage, and there's no way to predict your health at that time. So it's a good idea to hedge your gamble by buying $1,000 or $2,000 of monthly-benefit coverage through group plans and the same amount of permanent (noncancelable) coverage from one or more companies like these:

☐ Guardian Life, 201 Park Avenue South, New York, N.Y. 10003
☐ Monarch Life, 1250 State St., Springfield, Mass. 01101
☐ Provident Life and Accident, Fountain Square, Chattanooga, Tenn. 37402
☐ Paul Revere Life, 18 Chestnut St., Worcester, Mass. 01608
☐ Union Mutual Life, 2211 Congress St., Portland, Me. 04112
☐ William M. Mercer Inc., 222 South Riverside, Chicago, Ill. 60606;
   (800) 621-0366 (for A.M.A.-endorsed 12-month-exclusion coverage)

an umbrella topper. But check two or three of the general insurance brokers listed in your Yellow Pages before buying any coverage in your new community; one of those brokers may be willing to go out of his way to find you an umbrella policy as an inducement to let him write all your liability and property coverage.

The price of malpractice-insurance coverage depends, as you probably know, on your specialty and locale. I'm reluctant to make many more generalizations, because developments with regard to malpractice insurance coverage are occurring so rapidly that even generalities, to say nothing of specifics, are subject to considerable change between the time I write these words and the time you read them.

I will permit myself this observation, however: I'm not sure that the malpractice-premium problem is nearly as big as all the noise indicates. Many doctors in part-time practices and badly managed practices are hurting, to be sure, since they pay the same amount as the big earners for their policies. I think that's a serious problem. I do believe that the professor who sees a few patients on the side ought to be encouraged somehow to do so, not penalized with a full malpractice premium for a very small practice.

But I'm not addressing these remarks to professors or other part-time practitioners nor to people who are intent on managing their practices badly. Just the fact that you've read this book through this far seems evidence to me that you're a good candidate to run a well-managed practice, and that kind in 1976 usually paid less than 4 per cent of their production for malpractice insurance coverage and often paid less than 1 per cent.

If that's evidence of a crisis, then we've got a crisis. But even if you're a neurosurgeon, an orthopedist, or some other high-risk practitioner—even if you practice in New York or California or some other high-premium area and need to pay $10,000 to $25,000 for malpractice insurance—the odds are that you'll probably have more than $170,000 left for other practice expenses and your own compensation.

If you're a general surgeon, OB/Gyn specialist, or E.N.T. specialist, you won't do nearly as well, but that's because doctors in

*(Continued on page 281)*

**277**

FIGURE 21-5 ═══════════════════════════════════════════════

## A Roundup: The Insurance

Medical-management consultants—real ones, that is—never sell insurance or work with salespeople who do. But most of us do act as consultants in that area. Sometimes we help a client find the best price. More often, we look over his coverage and make suggestions. My own advice is summarized in this excerpt from a practice-survey report.

**Disability Coverage:** pays $1,000 per month till age 70 if disabled between ages 50 and 70 or for life if disabled before age 50. One-year elimination period. Premiums in group practice paid as a part of basic overhead. Typical premiums: $270 yearly at age 60-64, $130 at age 50-54; $140 at age 40-44; $80 under age 35. For details and an application write: William M. Mercer Inc., 222 South Riverside, Chicago, Ill. 60606

**Additional Disability Coverage:** either $1,000 or $2,000 per month of permanent (nongroup) protection from any of the leading disability-insurance companies [see address list in Figure 21-4]. Six-month elimination period. Payable for life in the event of total disability due to accident, till age 65 for disability due to sickness. Typical annual premium for $1,000 of coverage: $550 annually at age 45, $500 at age 35.

**In addition:** another $1,000 or $2,000 of group coverage through your county, state, or national society. Three-month exclusion. Typical premium: $200 per year at age 45. All such additional coverage to be treated as a chargeback to the doctor's compensation fund.

**Coverage for Assistants:** recommended in an amount not less than 10% of the total coverage for the most-insured doctor. Elimination period of 30 days. Check the doctors' insurers for special employee protection plans for garden-variety employees. Assistants' premiums to be included with basic overhead.

**Life Insurance:** pays $50,000 (or other sum, as agreed) as a part of the group-term life insurance plan adopted by a P.C. as an employee benefit. Not related to redemption of stock in the P.C. Thus, the company gets back its stock at book value, and the beneficiary is paid $50,000, free of capital gains tax, in a nonrelated transaction—tax-free, if ownership has been assigned so as to keep the insurance proceeds out of the estate. No key-man life insurance required, thus no purchase of life insurance with after-tax corporation or personal dollars.

**Additional Life Insurance Coverage:** Buy yearly renewable term life for the least expensive premium bid available. As you need less coverage, buy less. Some policies permit smaller amounts of coverage, as you wish, without penalty or any

## We Often Recommend

requirement of a new health examination. Some policies guarantee renewability to as much as age 100.

**Caveat Emptor: Cash-Value Life Insurance.** The premium outlay is three to seven times greater than that for guaranteed renewable term life. You must pay that price for about 20 years before the cash-value yearly premium equals the slowly rising premium for yearly renewable term. Term coverage does rise in price each year—but slowly. Cash-value coverage, which is marketed in a bewildering array of terminology, holds out the promise of something for nothing ("your money back"), which is more illusory than real. Salesmen earn lots more commissions by selling this kind than the term and are trained to counter all arguments against it. For that reason, what you read here will be branded as false (it is not), and you will probably buy what's best for the salesman, rather than what's best for you. Cash-value life insurance (whole life, ordinary life) has been described in Congressional testimony as "America's No. 1 consumer fraud." That goes double for so-called minimum-deposit insurance, which is cash-value coverage with a twist. That's the kind doctors end up buying.

**Example of Wise Coverage:** Doctor age 35: $50,000 of coverage through P.C. employee-benefit plan, $135 annually (deductible by the P.C.; $250,000 of coverage from personal funds, $677; total outlay for $300,000 of protection, $812. Wiser still, if the P.C. has few or no employees working over 1,000 hours a year: a full $300,000 of protection through the P.C. employee benefit plan.

**Coverage For Assistants:** required by I.R.S. with mixed support for its position by the courts. Best bet: Provide coverage in an amount equal to 10% of the coverage for doctors; for example, $5,000/$50,000. Premium depends on amount of coverage and age of each employee; $5,000: age 50, $87; age 40, $52; age 30, $41; age 25, $38.

**Overhead Insurance:** It doesn't cost a fortune ($550 yearly at age 45 for $5,000 monthly benefits under an A.M.A.-endorsed policy). O.K. if it pays what you expect. So we're not against it—nor are we enthusiastic about it. It's much like fire insurance: You'll never know how much it will actually pay till you've filed your claim. Premiums are tax-deductible. If in doubt, buy it. Get it from a plan endorsed by your county, state, or national medical society.

**Health Insurance:** Get major medical and excess-limits major medical. The assistant who does your claim forms can tell you which companies' policies are the best. Premiums are reimbursable by your corporation's health-care expense employee benefit plan.

FIGURE 21-6 ═══════════════════════════════════════════

## Some Good Sources of Financial
## Information and Advice

### MAGAZINES, NEWSLETTERS, AND NEWSPAPERS

☐ Better Homes and Gardens, $8 yearly, 1716 Locust St., Des Moines, Iowa 50336

☐ Changing Times, The Kiplinger Magazine, $9 yearly, Editors Park, Md. 20782

☐ Consumer Reports, $9.50 yearly, Consumers Union, Orangeburg, N.Y. 10962

☐ Growth Fund Guide, $45 yearly, Growth Fund Research Building, Yreka, Calif. 96097

☐ Medical Economics, free to certain physicians in private practice, $36 yearly to all others, Box 55, Oradell, N.J. 07649

☐ Medical World News, free to certain physicians in private practice, $25 yearly to all others, McGraw-Hill, Inc., 4530 West 77th St., Minneapolis, Minn. 55435

☐ Money, $14 yearly, Time, Inc., 541 North Fairbanks Ct., Chicago, Ill. 60611

☐ The New York Times, $145 yearly for delivery by mail (seven days), 229 West 43rd St., New York, N.Y. 10036

☐ United Mutual Fund Selector, $49 yearly, 212 Newbury St., Boston, Mass. 02116

☐ The Wall Street Journal, $45 yearly for delivery by mail, 200 Burnett Rd., Chicopee, Mass. 01021

Note: Prices are subject to change.

### BOOK CLUBS AND PUBLISHERS

☐ Books by U.S. News & World Report, Box 951, Hicksville, N.Y. 11802

☐ Chilton Book Company, Radnor, Pa. 19089

☐ Commerce Clearing House, Inc., 4025 West Peterson Ave., Chicago, Ill. 60646

☐ Conservative Book Club, 165 Huguenot St., New Rochelle, N.Y. 10801

☐ Dow Jones Books, Box 455, Chicopee, Mass. 01021

☐ The Executive Program, Riverside, N.J. 08075

☐ Farnsworth Publishing Company, Inc., 78 Randall Ave., Rockville Centre, N.Y. 11570

☐ Fortune Book Club, Camp Hill, Pa. 17012

☐ Foundation for Individual Enterprise, 415 Beneficial Bldg., Wilmington, Del. 19801

☐ The Hirsch Organization, Inc., 6 Deer Trail, Old Tappan, N.J. 07675

☐ Institute for Business Planning, Inc., Box 113, West Nyack, N.Y. 10994

☐ Investors Book Club, Riverside, N.J. 08075

☐ The McGraw-Hill Management Book Guild, Box 582, Hightstown, N.J. 08520

☐ Medical Economics Book Division, Oradell, N.J. 07649

those specialties don't produce or earn nearly as much as those in the high-risk group. A typical general surgeon pays 4-5 per cent of his production for malpractice coverage but still has more than $135,000 left for other overhead and his own compensation.

Across the country, most G.P.s and family practitioners pay less than 1 per cent of production, leaving them more than $135,000. Knowing the figures and knowing that there's at least a fair chance the whole malpractice crisis may be ended by Federal or state legislative action, I can't raise nearly as much interest in it as I do in matters like office location, layout, and staffing.

Of course, you do need to buy coverage, probably as much as your insurer will sell. Forget about going bare, at least until we see how badly hurt someone else is as a result of deliberately going without the insurance coverage. Judicial precedent suggests that the courts may undo the attempts by such a physician to dispose of his assets (through gifts to family members and the establishment of trust funds) and require liquidation of those assets in satisfaction of a malpractice award or slap a lien on the doctor that will take a significant portion of his earnings for years to come, whether he remains in private practice or works elsewhere, in or out of medicine. It could happen. Meantime, I suggest that you watch socioeconomic publications like Medical Economics and American Medical News for developments in the malpractice sector.

Since your family's financial security may depend on your life-insurance and malpractice-insurance protection, you need to pay special attention to those two coverages. But here's a rundown on the other kinds of insurance you need:

1. *Car insurance.* Developments in this field are occurring almost as rapidly as in the malpractice field, but, as I write these words, it still pays in most parts of the country to shop for coverage. The day will come, I suspect, when, to get auto insurance, you'll need to agree to buy homeowners and perhaps other kinds of insurance, too, from the same company. But for now, at least, you can still shop among various companies for auto insurance alone and, by so doing, save yourself some money.

In a study not long ago by the Pennsylvania Insurance Department, the cost of certain basic coverages by the highest-premium company was 226 per cent of the premium charged by the lowest-premium insurer. Among the lower-premium companies in that study were Federal Kemper, Home Insurance, Pacific Employers, United Services, Aetna Casualty, Travelers Indemnity, Volkswagen Insurance, City Insurance, Vigilant Insurance (also known as Sea Insurance), and Allstate.

When your car is two or three years old or as soon as you think you can self-insure its total replacement, drop collision coverage. Till that time, take the largest deductible offered by your company, probably $250.

Similarly, take the largest deductible offered for comprehensive coverage (fire, vandalism, theft). And do take uninsured-motorists coverage, even if you're not required by your state law to do so. Across the U.S., 15 to 20 per cent of all drivers carry no insurance, even in states where it's legally required. Alabama, Georgia, Louisiana, Mississippi, and Rhode Island have the largest number of uninsured drivers.

When you rent a car, you'd better take the $1.50-to-$2.50-a-day waiver of collision coverage, but don't even deal with a car-rental company that has supporting liability coverage of less than $100,000/$300,000/$25,000 as its limit for one person/limit for one accident/limit for property damage. The amount of such coverage is found in the small print on the rental form; check it before signing a car out.

2. *Disability insurance.* Avoid any policy that subtracts Social Security, workmen's compensation, or employer's sick-pay benefits, as well as policies that stop paying benefits once you're able to hold down *any* job. It's better to get a policy that defines disability as inability to function fully as a practicing physician, and better still is a definition that says you must be able to perform in your particular specialty.

Also, be sure the benefits continue at least through age 65 for both accident and sickness disability.

I often recommend $3,000 a month coverage in three policies—group coverage through a county, state, or specialty society plan, with an elimination period of either 30 or 60 days (usually 60); a noncancelable private policy through one of the major disability insurers (Guardian, Monarch, North American Company for Life & Health, Paul Revere, Provident Life, and Union Mutual, to name six of them), with an elimination period of either 90 or 120 days (usually 120); and the A.M.A.-endorsed coverage in the amount of $1,000 a month, like the other two, with a one-year elimination period.

Do get a waiver of premium in the event of disability, plus the right to purchase added protection without additional proof of insurability.

Let your professional corporation pay for and tax-deduct as a business expense all your disability-insurance premiums, but, except for that portion representing the first $100 of benefits per week (get the insurance man who sold you the private, noncancelable policy to give you a written breakdown of the premium), let the rest of the premiums of the three policies be recorded as additional taxable income to you. About half the money you thus report on your Form W-2 will be the tax you'll pay, but any benefits you receive should be completely free of income taxes. Remember: Employer-paid benefits are taxable, but benefits from a policy paid for by an individual are not taxable.

Also, when setting up your professional corporation retirement plan, see that there's a clause providing for a lump-sum distribution in the event of total disability. A U.S. District Court ruled not long ago that such a clause makes the distribution a nontaxable health benefit, rather than taxable retirement pay. Future judicial or legislative action may take away that opportunity, but at least for now the clause is a worthy addition to your retirement plan.

3. *Health insurance.* Let your professional corporation pay for it, along the lines we discussed in Chapters 16 and 17—Blue Cross, Blue Shield, major medical, and excess-limits major medical. And get the whole ball of wax.

4. *House insurance.* To collect fully, you've got to have your place insured for at least 80 per cent of its replacement value. So you've got to review this coverage annually. It can pay to shop around (independent agents often sell at higher prices than do one-insurer salesmen), but it can be just as important to take as big a deductible as the company allows (often $500).

Buy the best comprehensive coverage you can find, but be warned that it doesn't cover everything. You have to ask about a special schedule for valuable coins, stamps, works of art, golf clubs and other valuable sporting equipment, cameras, and jewelry.

Also remember that homeowners policies do not cover sewer backups, tidal waves, or high water; protection against those events is available through flood insurance, sold by the 120 companies that belong to the National Flood Insurance Association.

5. *Office insurance.* In many parts of the country, doctors buy their office-liability protection from the same insurer who sells them malpractice coverage, usually at a favorable premium rate. Several inexpensive riders and endorsements are worth adding to the basic coverage. I recommend loss-of-rent protection (if you own the office), replacement of leasehold improvements (if you're a tenant), paper-and-records protection (it pays the cost of reconstructing charts), accounts-receivable protection (unless you're on computer billing, in which case you may not need it), business-interruption coverage, fine-arts protection (if you have valuable art in the office), and, often in a supplementary policy, nonownership auto coverage in the amounts of $100,000/$300,000/$50,000.

Finally, covering both your financial present and future:
● *Your practice management.* A lot of your older colleagues have lost sight of a basic and obvious truth: A physician's career is easily the soundest and best investment he'll ever make. You'll work hard in private practice, but you'll get enormous satisfaction from it. As Dr. Bodner discovered, there's no greater wealth than that. And the pay is pretty good, too.

To further your career and to review some of the basic points covered in this book, let's close by taking a look at my 10 key rules of practice management:

1. Choose the specialty that captures your interest. God knows the world needs pediatricians. But lots of pediatricians eventually come to believe they'd make better internists. Or radiologists. Or anesthesiologists.

2. Be the best you can be in your specialty. It's hard to take *too* much continuing education.

3. Go where your services are needed.

4. Never skimp on workrooms. You'll need at least one or two more examining rooms than you'll get.

5. Hire only the help you need, but hire the best people you can find. The right way to keep overhead in check is to increase productivity, not to buy cheap.

6. Treat your staff as a team, and you be the player-coach. Everyone likes to be near a superstar. He's inspirational.

7. Delegate, delegate, delegate. You're crazy to do work you can usefully and legally delegate to an assistant.

8. Constantly plan ahead for more office, more staff, more equipment. Use your monthly management-report worksheet.

9. Always wear a white hat. Your mother loves you. Why shouldn't Main Street?

10. Never forget: Better practice management is often the better alternative to a fee increase.

Don't come bragging to me that you're a lousy businessman. If you really have your patients' interests at heart, you'll work hard at being a good businessman, a good administrator, and a good manager of your practice.

Before any client of mine increases his fees, I ask him to convince himself that he can't find a way to increase patient volume, to increase his practice's productivity, to increase gross practice income. And I *don't* mean by running patients through the office in assembly-line fashion or by beating everyone over the head for money. Often more can be delegated to your assistants, with proper planning and training. They can handle more phone calls, take the initial patient histories, close gaps in the appointment schedule, get the monthly bills out on time, eliminate the backlog of health-insurance forms, and offer patients a chance to pay at the time of service by using charge slips and superbills.

Also, I suggest that you first review your personal finances. I've seen windfalls of $40,000 and more result instantly by simply taking the tax-free cash values built up in high-priced life insurance and replacing it with yearly renewable term and by selling off the hopeless losers among common stocks and mutual funds.

Sometimes existing loans and debts can be recast by sending a frank letter to creditors, requesting a three-month moratorium, to be followed by a series of equal monthly payments. Loans that can't be recast can often be paid off advantageously by a debt-consolidation loan—preferably a personal loan from a commercial bank or savings institution.

And sometimes I find that a doctor-client needs to wake up to the fact that he's living well beyond his means. When that's the case, the basic problem, as in alcoholism, is to admit that a problem exists and to express an earnest willingness to solve it. Then the credit cards can be locked away, and payment can be made only with currency. Meals and drinks out are reduced, as are other expensive leisure activities. Plans are delayed for buying a new car or new furnishings. The vacation home may have to go. Why buy what you can't afford?

Don't get me wrong. Like my client Dr. Bodner, you have a right to the good life, the country club, the new Mercedes. I never begrudged him any of those things. The fact that he's put away relatively little over the span of his career is perhaps less a reflection on him than on Congress, which only in recent years got around to passing laws that allow doctors, lawyers, and other professional people to accumulate enough funds through their retirement plans to provide a base of financial security. Anyway, Dr. Bodner is a successful professional man, a major asset to his community, and he deserves to live comfortably—at least as much as any banker or executive or professional athlete in town.

"Just tell them," Dr. Bodner suggested when I asked him for permission to use his story in this book, "not to be in such an all-fired rush to live well. First, get your practice humming. And be one hell of a doctor. You do those two things, and you won't have to worry about the good life. It naturally follows."

Believe it.